Symptoms and Diagnosis

A Storytelling Medical Book That May Save Your Life

Nabin Sapkota, MD

Symptoms and Diagnosis

Printed in the USA

Copyright © 2016 by Nabin Sapkota, MD

ISBN-13: 978-0-9826965-2-1
ISBN-10: 0-9826965-2-3

MedTale Publishing
Omaha, NE
www.symptomsdiagnosisbook.com

Disclaimer: The information presented in this book is for
educational purposes only. It should not, in any way, be
considered medical advice. If you need any specific advice
about your own symptoms, visit your doctor. You have a
unique story of your own illness, and your doctor can treat you
only after considering your unique circumstances.

This book is dedicated to all of my patients and their families.

Contents

Acknowledgments

A busy medical doctor with a full-time practice cannot write and publish a book like this without help from a team of publishing experts. I am truly indebted to those experts for shaping my ideas and intentions in this book.

This book would not have been possible without the enthusiasm, encouragement, and guidance of my literary agent, Rita Rosenkranz. With her many years of experience in publishing, she has molded this project into an actual, marketable book.

Elana Seplow-Jolley is the best editor one could ask for as a doctor working on a book for patients. She honed my voice and made my advice more user friendly. I would like to thank her for working tirelessly to make this book better, little by little, one revision at a time.

My cover designer, Benjamin Martin, is a talented artist and visionary designer. His brilliant cover art brought my ideas to life. I would like to thank him for working so patiently with my team to make sure everyone was on board with his incredible designs.

I would like to thank my teachers at Cook County Hospital, Chicago, for teaching me the importance of patient stories. I especially remember the words of Dr. Brendan Riley, the chairman of medicine at the time, who showed us that by listening more closely to patients, we can reach more accurate diagnoses. His words planted the seeds of this book ten years ago.

Finally, I would like to thank my wife, Rashmi, for encouraging me to find time for writing even when it seemed like twenty-four hours were not enough for a day. Without her by my side keeping it all together, it would not have been possible to balance a medical practice, an active family, and writing.

Foreword

Brian J. Bossard, MD

In a world that becomes increasingly dependent on technology every day, communication runs the risk of becoming evermore remote and more virtual. We text, we tweet, and we chat—the Internet and technology have changed the way we connect with each other. Connectivity is measured in terms of bandwidth and megabytes of data, not in the amount of time we spend talking to each other or touching one another. In the pages of this book, Dr. Nabin Sapkota provides us with a refreshing reminder of the importance of our feelings, our observations, and our personal interactions.

This is a book written from a fascinating perspective by a unique physician with a unique background. A native of Nepal, Nabin Sapkota excelled in his undergraduate work in Kathmandu. He received a scholarship to study medicine in neighboring China, although he did not speak the language. After a year of Mandarin, Nabin completed his medical degree in Shanghai, China. Dr. Sapkota then pursued medical residency training in Chicago at Cook County Hospital.

I have known Dr. Sapkota for many years and have had the pleasure of working with him to open a new medical practice in a rural community. His expansive expertise in the field of acute care and hospital-based internal medicine informs every aspect of his daily work and every chapter of this book. The case histories presented here are drawn from circumstances he has encountered on a daily basis in his medical practice. As a doctor and a teacher, Dr. Sapkota excels in distilling complex medical issues down to fundamental, approachable concepts. His clever approach to contextualizing each case with an introductory teaching point reflects his passion for education and compassion for his patients. The lessons in this book are mandatory reading for every medical student, nursing student, and physician's assistant, but all readers will find this book engaging and educational, regardless of their level of medical knowledge or understanding of health-care jargon. Doctors, nurses, trainees, and patients alike must learn to see medicine through the eyes of the patient.

Dr. Nabin Sapkota is an accomplished internal-medicine physician, a gifted storyteller, and a devoted and passionate educator. His lifelong pursuit of seeing medical practice through the eyes of his patients and of helping his patients better understand his perspective as a medical doctor has empowered his patients for years. Now it can empower you as well. This book unlocks the mysteries of medicine, chapter by understandable and engaging chapter. If you are interested in unraveling the mystery of how your body works, of why your body makes you feel the way that you feel, of what your body is trying to tell you, read on.

Brian J. Bossard, MD

Introduction

Using This Book

When people hear about a disease, their first question is usually, "What are the symptoms?" In reality, symptoms are personal experiences patients have when they are sick. Patients often have difficulty describing these signs in concrete terms. That's why it's crucial to ask what symptoms mean when they manifest in a specific patient rather than what medical condition the symptoms match.

While medical expertise is the most powerful tool a doctor wields to treat a patient under his or her care, its effectiveness is greatly increased when that medical knowledge is transferred from doctor to patient. Patients also have a unique store of knowledge that grows more powerful when transferred to doctors: the experience of their own symptoms. When doctors and patients transfer their knowledge to each other by listening and communicating, everyone wins. That's why it's so important for patients to be conscious of their experience of symptoms and to describe them to their doctors as only they can.

Since it's often difficult to listen to your body without understanding what it's telling you, I want to help you communicate better with your doctor and with your own body by teaching you the proper way to analyze any symptom you experience. When you understand what actually happens deep inside your organs and tissues, you are able to make sense of what your body is trying to say. You can then help your doctor predict the correct diagnosis without having to define your symptoms. This skill can save your life by alerting you and your doctor to a medical emergency, even when you have atypical or unusual symptoms. *Symptoms and Diagnosis* empowers you by telling the stories of real patients in life-threatening situations whose lives were saved by listening to their bodies when they felt sick and connecting what they were feeling to what was happening to their bodies.

You don't need to be a doctor to understand *Symptoms and Diagnosis*, but this book is structured around a tried-and-true medical-school teaching principle: teaching by example and using patient stories to convey lifesaving information. The twenty stories featured in this book cover most organ systems and represent the majority of common diseases and conditions that are seen in most acute-care hospitals in the United States. Each story describes how a patient felt at the onset of symptoms and connects it to what actually happened inside the organs. This book is also designed to illuminate how your body works and what happens when you get sick.

While each chapter is dedicated to a particular organ system, *Symptoms and Diagnosis* is constructed to thoroughly familiarize you with the right way to analyze any symptoms you may experience. I recommend reading the entire book to broaden your understanding of how your body works. Once you've got the bigger picture, you can revisit a particular organ system by going back to the story relating to that organ. For example, if you want to learn more about infection and fevers, you can reread chapter 2; if you want to learn more about heart attacks, you can reread chapter 3.

Each story is followed by a discussion of the key medical topics encountered in the story. The discussion is divided into two parts. The first part gives you some important information to help you learn the basic approach to put symptoms in the right context. The second part discusses the actual organ systems involved in the story and tells you what happens to them when you get sick. By using each story as a reference, not only will you learn how the symptoms of a particular disease present in a particular patient, but you will also learn the method of analyzing symptoms in the proper way.

1. When Symptoms Attack

How Describing Symptoms Saved Aaron's Life

The accurate description of the onset of your symptoms is sometimes more important than the actual manifestation.

For Aaron, the morning started off like any other. As he walked to his car, little did he know that in the next few hours, he would have to fight for his life. A fifty-five-year-old nonsmoker who led an active lifestyle, Aaron watched what he ate and tried to maintain a good weight. He didn't particularly like going to the doctor, so he tried his best to lead a healthy life. One day he woke up refreshed and ready to face the day. He ate breakfast, said good-bye to his wife and son, and walked out of the house. Halfway to his car, Aaron stumbled slightly and stopped dead in his tracks. He fell to the ground. He felt as if all the life had been sucked out of his body in a single instant. He had never experienced anything like this before. As his wife and son ran to him, he tried to get up from the ground but found that he couldn't. To his horror, he realized his legs were fluttering instead of moving normally. It felt like all the muscles in his body had been suddenly cut loose from his brain, and it took all of his energy to stay aware of how he felt.

Aaron could sense a tremendous amount of stress in his body, which he tried very hard to control. At first he felt as though he did not have sufficient strength to support his body, much less control it, but he kept trying. He struggled to stop his arms and legs from moving involuntarily. When his efforts seemed to produce some small results, he persisted, pushing even harder. He still had some control of his body, he realized. He just needed to push harder to regain control.

Within the next five minutes, Aaron managed not only to stop his limbs from fluttering but also to move them. He found he could push himself up from the ground and hold out his arms for support. With his son firmly grasping his right hand, and his wife holding his left, he managed to get inside the house and lie down on the couch. His son called 911. By the time paramedics arrived to take him to the nearby rural hospital, Aaron felt much better. He was still very weak, but he was almost in complete control of his body. He wasn't in pain, and he was breathing easily. On the way to the hospital, he thought about his family. He didn't know what had happened back in his driveway, but he knew he needed to find out. He loved his family, and he wasn't ready to die.

At the hospital, Aaron got more questions than answers. He tried to answer questions from doctors and orderlies faithfully in the hope of helping reach a diagnosis. After several x-rays, a CAT scan, heart monitoring, and blood tests, Aaron met his doctor. The look on his doctor's face made Aaron nervous, but doctors always made Aaron nervous.

"So far, everything looks good," said the doctor. "It appears that you had a seizure, but we haven't yet found any specific cause for the seizure. Then again, we can't always locate the cause of a seizure."

A seizure? He had absolutely no idea what a seizure was. He had never needed—or wanted—to know. All his life, he had actively avoided learning anything about diseases and their symptoms. They reminded him of his own mortality. But things were different now. The doctor explained that when you had the seizure, the part of your brain that is normally under your control—the part that allowed Aaron to nod his head as the doctor spoke—was seized.

Neurological (nerve) events, the doctor explained, could happen instantly, but the end results could be complex. When a nerve connected to an organ was cut off, the organ could still function because of a second nerve branch that led to the organ from a different source. The brain was made up of millions of these nerve cells that networked with each other. If a nerve was cut off, another could take over. Millions of interconnected nerve cells firing without control could produce bizarre symptoms.

The doctor paused for a moment, frowning at Aaron's chart. He asked a nurse to check Aaron's blood pressure one more time. It was 91/44.

The doctor excused himself, but the nurse remained by Aaron's side. His blood pressure, she told him, was a little lower than the doctor would have liked. Normal blood pressure was 100–120/60–80. The first number stood for the pressure level at which the heart pumped out blood to the body. The lower number described the pressure level present when the heart relaxed, drawing in blood. That in-and-out contraction and relaxation made up Aaron's heartbeat. Blood pressure could fluctuate depending on a person's mood, level of anxiety, and level of activity. Aaron knew that having high blood pressure could lead to a heart attack or stroke (he'd seen the blood-pressure medication ads on TV), but what could low blood pressure do? The nurse assured Aaron that low blood pressure was usually nothing to worry about—some people naturally had lower blood pressure than others.

As Aaron tried to make sense of this new information, the doctor returned. Aaron's blood pressure was unusually low for someone who had just had a seizure. "Something about your case makes me uncomfortable," he said. "I think it's time for you to see a specialist at the regional medical center. They can run more tests and try to figure out exactly what happened to you."

At the larger regional ICU with his wife and son, Aaron met another doctor. As the new doctor reviewed Aaron's chart, he began asking questions, pressing Aaron for greater detail than the first doctor had. Aaron suddenly realized he wanted the doctor to ask as many questions as he needed to get to the right diagnosis. He had no idea that this realization would turn out to be a lifesaving one.

He started at the very beginning, telling the doctor everything that had happened to him from the moment he walked out of his house. He described his garage and how he had been walking toward his car when he had the seizure.

"I don't just want to hear that you had a seizure," the doctor interrupted. "I want to know exactly how you felt as your symptoms set in."

Inspired by the doctor's persistent questioning, Aaron thought deeply, trying to remember exactly how he had felt. In the rush, full of anxiety, he had almost forgotten the initial experience. He had described his attack objectively, leaving out his own feelings. As he thought harder about his attack, a memory came flooding back to Aaron. He recalled how he had felt not entirely out of control but enervated in an instant, as if a switch had been flipped inside of him. He had felt light-headed and weak, unable to even stand. Pained, he remembered the deep helplessness that had washed over him as his wife and son watched him. It had felt like an eternity before he slowly regained strength and his muscles had begun to tense as he wanted them to. These were words he hadn't spoken aloud before.

As he spoke about how he felt, he realized there was something wrong with his first doctor's logic. If he had, in fact, experienced a seizure, and he had not been able to send commands from his brain to his body, then how had he even been able to regain incremental amounts of strength by concentrating on controlling his fluttering limbs? With a jolt of realization, Aaron met the doctor's gaze. He saw that same realization reflected back at him.

"I don't think you had a seizure," Aaron's doctor said. "To have the kind of seizure that moves all your limbs, it must involve a large part of the brain. A spark would have to start somewhere in the brain and spread to the rest of the brain. The nerves in a large part of your brain had to be firing without any control for you to go down and start shaking involuntarily. That doesn't sound like what you described."

Aaron nodded. He hadn't felt completely out of control, just out of energy. Yes, he had to expend extra effort to think, but he was still able to concentrate all his available energy to retake control of his legs.

"The flipping of a switch," the doctor repeated. "Yes, of course. That sounds like a vascular event." A vascular event, the doctor explained, was an event that cut off the blood supply to an organ, a system of organs, or the whole body. Blood was essential to sustain the lives of cells, organs, tissues, and a person as a whole. "When the blood supply is cut off, symptoms appear instantaneously. If you cut off the blood supply to an organ, then that organ will stop working right away. Switch off the blood going to your heart muscles, and you get a heart attack. Cut off the blood supply to your right leg, and you have a right lower limb ischemia on your hands. Switch off the blood supply to your gut, and you get a gut attack called bowel ischemia. No matter what symptoms you have, if they occur in an instant, as if at the flip of a switch, you need to consider a vascular event first."

Based on his weakness, the doctor explained, it seemed like Aaron had lost function of his whole body. It was possible that the blood supply to Aaron's whole body had been compromised. Aaron was about to ask how that could happen when a nurse popped her head into the examination room. Aaron's blood pressure, she said, was still dropping.

"A loss of blood supply and low blood pressure?" Aaron's doctor nodded. "That makes sense. Your whole body's blood supply must indeed have been cut off." But how? Was Aaron's heart not pumping enough blood? Was the blood supply cut off after it came out of the heart? It was possible that something had happened in Aaron's chest, immediately upward in the neck, at the level of his heart or at one of the major arteries carrying blood to the rest of the body. Without further delay, the doctor ordered a CAT scan of Aaron's chest. All Aaron's questions were about to be answered—and not a moment too soon.

The CAT scan showed that there was a major tear in the big artery that came directly out of Aaron's heart— an aortic dissection. That single tear extended into Aaron's neck and was blocking most of the blood going into his brain. Ever since his attack, Aaron had been surviving solely on the blood that was escaping through that colossal blockage, and if he didn't act fast, he was essentially living on borrowed time. There wasn't a minute to lose; the mortality rate for sufferers was 10 percent for every hour lost before surgery. Only four hours after the attack, Aaron had a 40 percent chance of dying.

He was taken into surgery, given a shot, and then it was all a dream. He woke up in his room in the ICU. His body ached, and he found that his chest was bandaged.

Another doctor stood beside his bed, checking his heart monitor. Aaron shook his head groggily and asked what time it was. The doctor smiled. Aaron had survived a very difficult five-hour surgery in which the tear had been fixed. "It's late. How are you feeling?" the doctor asked.

Aaron felt like he was in a dream all over again. His recovery began slowly but healthily. Over the next few days, he reflected on the timely conversation that had saved his life. There were certain aspects of his symptoms that only he could see. By describing his experience of his symptoms fully, he had given his doctor the cipher to interpret his symptoms. He was glad he had met that second doctor. When the first doctor had described seizure symptoms, Aaron had sensed they didn't match the symptoms he had experienced, but he had lacked confidence in his instincts and his own medical knowledge to tell the doctor what he had felt. Later he learned that this was not an uncommon problem for patients with little medical knowledge.

When he returned home, he began reading up on vascular events in medical journals and online. He couldn't help feeling as though he could have targeted his ailment earlier if he'd known his body better. He also couldn't help wanting a more accessible source of medical knowledge. Medical knowledge, he realized, was lifesaving, not anxiety producing.

Teaching Points

Basic Approach: The Onset of Symptoms

When you get sick, every small detail of your symptoms can make a huge difference in your diagnosis. According to most studies, doctors make one wrong diagnosis in every eight patients they see. The most important factor in the incorrect diagnosis is miscommunication. Doctors have been trained to improve their communication skills for decades using countless books, trainings, conferences and seminars, but your doctor constitutes only half of the communication equation. It's important to educate yourself and to pay attention to what your body is telling you. In doing so, you'll help your doctor save your life. When you get sick, it is very important to note how your symptoms started. When you have pain or discomfort, it is easy to focus on the symptom itself and not to notice the circumstances in which it started. The onset of symptoms is one of the most critical pieces of information that affects the line of diagnostic thinking.

Unfortunately, most of the information available to patients in books and health magazines and on TV and the Internet focuses on textbook disease symptoms, often neglecting smaller, subtler details that can crucially change the course of a diagnosis.

As in Aaron's case, the details of the onset of your symptoms can sometimes be more important than the actual descriptions of them. When you or your loved one starts to get sick, try to note exactly how the symptoms started. Take out your journal or your smartphone and make note of the exact time, place, and event that happened before you or your loved one got sick.

Here are some of the things about your symptoms that might hold the key to the correct diagnosis:

1. What exactly were you doing when your symptoms started? Were you sitting up, lying down, standing, talking, eating, sleeping, working on the computer, watching a movie or just resting comfortably? Remember you increase your chances of getting the right diagnosis by describing the circumstances around the onset of your symptoms in as much detail as you are able.

2. What was the first thing that happened? You may have felt a little dizzy or light-headed before you started having pain in your chest. It is often easy to focus on chest pain and to not even recall the sudden onset of slight dizziness that happened just before the chest pain started. That information would have alerted your doctor to a critical lifesaving diagnosis. Many people are alarmed when they have chest pain, but they don't always think much of a little light-headedness. When you get sick, try not to focus only on the dominant symptom, overwhelming as it may be. Try to notice and write down the first unusual thing that happened to you before you developed the main symptom.

3. How fast did the symptom develop? As Aaron's case illustrates, the exact timing of a symptom can provide information that can match that symptom with a completely different system of organs. If you can note the exact time it took to develop your symptom, your doctor can associate it with the right organ system and start following the correct diagnostic thread. Did the symptom occur within a fraction of a second, within a few seconds, within a minute, within a few minutes, within an hour, or within a few hours?

In an ideal world, you need not worry about these things; it is the doctor's job to establish a relationship by asking you questions to get every single detail of your symptom from you. In reality, no relationship is perfect. The doctor isn't always able to get all the important details from the patient.

Sometimes only you can provide these details, by being proactive and learning what is important. When you note all the minor details and communicate them clearly to your doctor, you do not have to be at the mercy of the doctor's communication skills. You can make sure your doctor has the right information to make the correct diagnosis. That is the first step to becoming an empowered patient.

The onset of your symptoms is one of the most important clues in deciphering your symptoms. There are other details about your symptoms that also play very important roles. You will learn about those in the subsequent chapters.

Organ System: Vascular

Now, let's review the basic knowledge of the organ systems we encountered in this story. Aortic dissection was the final diagnosis in the story. To get to the right diagnosis, symptoms must be first placed in the right organ system. Here the organ was a major blood vessel, the aorta, and the organ system was the vascular system. The first doctor's diagnosis of a seizure would have put the malfunctioning organ in the brain and the organ system as the nervous system.

How do these two systems work? And how does the onset of symptoms for each differ? You may have a tendency to associate certain symptoms with a certain disease, but symptoms, as we've seen, can be deceptive. The same symptom with a minor difference in detail can originate from a completely different disease from a completely different organ. For example, you may have chest pain from any of the organs that reside inside your chest. Each of those organs belongs to a different organ system and can have completely different diagnostic implications. The details of the chest pain help the doctor decide which diagnosis to pursue.

Let's explore the vascular system. The vascular system is our body's basic plumbing system for blood flow. Blood comes out of the left side of the heart, goes to all parts of the body, and returns to the right side of the heart. From the right side of the heart, it goes to the lungs, where it captures oxygen from the air we breathe

15

in. The fresh blood then goes back to the left side of the heart to be pumped into the rest of the body. The system of vessels that allows the blood to circulate this way makes up the vascular system. The vascular system has two major types of blood vessels: arteries and veins. Arteries are the vessels that carry the high-pressured blood out of the heart. They are made of thick walls to withstand this pressure. Veins are the thin-walled blood vessels that drain blood out of the organs and let it flow passively back into the heart.

In Aaron's case, the problem was caused by the high-blood-pressure system. For the low-pressure system, take a look at chapter 14. The high-pressure system starts as a large thick-walled vessel that carries all the blood out from the heart. This main supply line is called the aorta. It then divides into major branches to supply blood to major organs. As the branches move away from the heart, they further divide into a system of smaller branches and supply blood to the whole body.

When a branch of the artery gets obstructed, there is immediate loss of blood supply to the organs supplied by that branch and its sub-branches. When the onset of symptoms is rapid, we need to think about the vascular system. Aaron had a sudden-onset loss of blood supply to his whole body that resulted in his collapse. He was lucky to survive because the obstruction was incomplete and some blood was still flowing out. His problem lay in the aorta and therefore involved his whole body. A sudden loss of blood supply to the leg causes leg ischemia (for more on ischemia, see chapter 15). A sudden loss of blood supply to the heart causes heart attack (for more on heart attacks, see chapter 3).

Aortic dissection happens when the wall of the aorta gets damaged. The high-pressured blood then penetrates the wall of the aorta and blood rushes into a gap between the layers of the wall. The blood inside the wall layers pushes inward and narrows the lumen of the aorta. When a large amount of blood rushes into the wall layers, it can completely obstruct the main lumen or one of the main branches coming out of the aorta. Sometimes the pressure between the wall layers can get so high that it can rupture the aorta, causing immediate death. The onset of symptoms is always very rapid with aortic dissection. The most common symptom is a crushing, sudden-onset pain in the chest, but not all patients have the classic pain described in the textbooks. Any abrupt onset symptom that suggests major changes in blood supply should make you think about your diagnosis. Since the neurological system consists of your brain and all the nerves in your body, acting as your body's command and control center, it is very complex. The onset of nervous system diseases can likewise be variable and complicated. We will discuss the neurological system further in chapter 6 and chapter 7.

2. Listen to Your Body

How Sophie's Body Turned on Her When She Ignored Her Symptoms

It's important to listen to your body when it sends distress signals. Ignoring them can make them much worse.

Sophia had always been a morning person, but on one particular day she struggled to wake up and get out of bed. She didn't feel like herself. Usually she was full of energy in the morning, excited to start the day and head off to school. A middle-school math teacher, Sophia loved her job. She gently pushed her students to believe in themselves and helped them achieve more than they thought possible.

For a fleeting moment, Sophia felt as if her body was telling her that something bad was coming, but Sophia brushed the feeling aside and headed to work. She always cared about the well-being of others—her husband, her students, and her coworkers—more than she cared for her own. In class, despite feeling a slow tension building up in her body, as if every muscle were tightening up to defensively fight something off, she pushed herself to stay busy and act as though she felt perfectly fine. Not one of her coworkers suspected that Sophia was actually completely exhausted. Neither they nor Sophia knew she was at the beginning of a life-threatening battle.

By third period, the tension in Sophia's muscles was growing stronger by the minute, gradually translating into pain that could not be ignored. Sophia felt the pain all over her body, but it was most noticeable on the left side of her lower back. By lunchtime, she found she had completely lost her appetite. The cafeteria was serving her favorite meal—spaghetti with meatballs—but the smell of the meatballs made her feel sick. All she could do was finish a bottle of apple juice, even though her mouth was dry. A wave of nausea swept over her, and she ran to the bathroom, hoping to get whatever bug she had out of her system. When nothing came up but a dry heave, she went to her next class, resolving not to eat or drink anything for the rest of the day in case she might feel sick again—the last thing she wanted to do was appear sick to her students and coworkers.

By the afternoon, Sophia had developed a fever, but she still pushed herself to finish the school day. When she got home, she climbed directly into bed, exhausted. Acting as though she felt normal and healthy seemed to have taken an enormous amount of energy. She was right; her body was completely exhausted. She was too weak to stand, and her fever climbed. She felt cold and hot at the same time, shivering and sweating by turns under her comforter. She realized she had to get her fever down, but as she tried to stand up to walk to her medicine cabinet for some Tylenol, she almost fainted. As she slowly crawled back into bed, Sophia realized that her life was in real danger. It was time to admit that she wasn't fine. She called her husband at work, and he left immediately—not a moment too soon.

When he arrived home, Sophia's husband immediately called 911. He was alarmed at the state in which he had found Sophia. Her face was pale, her eyes appeared sunken, and her arms and legs felt cold and clammy to the touch. She was too weak to even speak clearly. He was afraid she would die.

Sophia was rushed to the emergency room, where a doctor told Sophia's husband that his wife was in a state of shock—her body was crashing, struggling to stay alive. Technically, the doctor explained, the body went into a state of shock when it was under so much stress that it was unable to sustain normal blood circulation. Of course the exact symptoms of shock vary from person to person—shock is usually a symptom of a larger problem—but the outcome would always be the same: a fight, a struggle, a loss, and a crash. Sophia must have been exhausted all day. She should have listened to her body. The next step, the doctor explained, would be to determine why Sophia was in shock.

The doctor showed Sophia's husband her chart. Sophia's blood pressure was 60/35. Normally a person's blood-pressure range was 100–120/60–80. Blood pressure, the doctor explained, was measured in milliliters of mercury. A pressure of 120 meant that the pressure had the capacity to raise a column of mercury up to a height of 120 milliliters against gravity. As her heart pumped blood, it was only able to generate a force equal to a column of 60 milliliters of mercury instead of the 120 it normally produced. In other words, her heart was so weak that it was only able to produce half the normal force. When Sophia's heart muscles relaxed, the pressure dropped down to a very low level of thirty-five milliliters of mercury. To compensate for the low pressure, her heart was beating very fast: 130 beats per minute.

"But why?" Sophia's husband asked. "Did Sophia have a heart attack?"

"That's a good question," the doctor replied, nodding his head. "But a weakly beating heart does not always mean that the heart is the problem. It means that the heart is not pumping enough blood—a problem that can occur for three different reasons."

The first cause, the doctor explained, could be actual weakness of the heart muscle. The heart was simply a pump that sent blood to the rest of the body. In this case, the problem would be the actual failure of the pump.

The second cause could be a deficiency of blood in the system. In that case, the pump would be fine, but it would not have enough blood to pump. As the blood returned to the heart, it would not fill it up properly. The half-full pump would not be able to pump out blood with the required force to push it far enough to circulate effectively throughout the body.

The third and last cause could be an increased demand for blood. Under certain conditions, more blood vessels opened up in the body as the demand for blood increased in different struggling organs. With too many of these new channels, the circulating blood volume would decrease. It would no longer be able to fill up the heart completely when it returned.

The doctor asked Sophia's husband when Sophia had started to get sick, as Sophia was now too weak to even get out a sentence. With a time line, the doctor could make some educated guesses about what had happened. If Sophia's attack came on instantly, she could have had a massive heart attack or a blood clot that would cause actual weakness in her heart muscles. If it happened quickly but not instantly, Sophia could be bleeding internally, resulting in too little blood in her body. If her symptoms had developed in more than a few hours or a few days, the attack could stem from an infection. The infection could put strain on different organs, resulting in high demand for blood.

Unfortunately, Sophia's husband had no idea that his wife had been sick before she had called. She hadn't said anything in the morning. By the time he had found her at home in bed that afternoon, she was too weak to talk. He called the school to ask if anyone had noticed Sophia flagging or exhibiting signs of illness. Sophia had behaved just as usual, he was told, with focus and cheerful enthusiasm. Her coworkers were shocked to hear that something was wrong. One colleague mentioned that she had noticed Sophia hadn't eaten lunch, but otherwise, no one could recall any other sign. Sophia had acted as if nothing was wrong.

The doctor had no clues to work from except for Sophia's fever (usually, though not always, fever means infection), but he knew he couldn't wait to get the diagnosis of infection-related shock confirmed before starting a course of treatment. The key to a diagnosis lay in Sophia's experience of her symptoms, but Sophia couldn't tell him her story. As an ER doctor, he knew that most lifesaving decisions were based on hunches or judgment calls, despite advanced medical technology. Time lost waiting for test results could be the difference between life and death, so he ordered blood tests and began a course of treatment. An infusion of two liters of saline solution was injected into Sophia's veins—the appropriate treatment for shock resulting from low blood volume and increased demand for blood.

The doctor knew that if Sophia had a serious infection with a high fever, her body would have lost water from evaporation. Infection would also have caused her appetite to go down, resulting in decreased water intake, as well as nausea and vomiting, resulting in further water loss. As blood is 60 percent water, loss of water means loss of blood volume.

The doctor also knew that infection could increase the demand for blood. Anytime a germ invaded the body, the immune system worked very hard to fight it off. Much of the immune system's defenses lay in the bloodstream. As the body detected invading germs, it produced certain chemicals that served to jumpstart the immune system. Some of those chemicals worked to open up more blood vessels to allow more blood, and therefore more fighter cells, to flow into the infected organ. As the infection grew worse, a surplus of those chemicals could overwhelm the body by opening up too many new channels for blood flow. Infusing the right kind of saline solution directly into Sophia's veins could increase the amount of blood volume needed to offset both these changes. But would it work?

It did. Sophia's blood pressure rose to 85/55, and her condition began to stabilize. Now the doctor could afford to wait to examine Sophia's blood-test results, which, it turned out, were not good. Sophia had high levels of toxic waste in her blood—such high levels, in fact, that her kidneys were not functioning properly. Could she be experiencing kidney failure? The answer lay in the blood tests.

The doctor had ordered tests for two different types of toxic-waste levels: blood urea nitrogen (BUN) and creatinine (Cr). BUN, he knew, was composed of several nitrogen compounds that formed when proteins in the body broke down. Cr was a compound specifically formed by the breakdown of muscles. The body produced these waste materials during normal chemical processes. Healthy kidneys filtered out these wastes from the blood and released them in urine.

If a patient's kidneys failed, these toxins accumulated in the blood. The levels of these toxins would give an indirect estimate of kidney function as measured by their ability to filter blood in milliliters per minute. Normal kidney function estimates would be equal to or greater than sixty. Kidney function estimates less than ten indicated total renal failures. Sophie's kidney function was estimated to be less than ten. The doctor remained calm, however.

Sophia's blood pressure continued to improve. As it did, Sophia grew more alert and able to speak in a low, soft voice. The doctor rushed to her bedside, hoping to get the crucial information that only she could provide. Struggling to speak, Sophia described how she had felt during the day—her exhaustion, nausea, and muscle

23

tension in the lower-left quadrant of her back. The doctor realized there was a very good possibility that Sophia had an infection in her left kidney. A urine test would be able to confirm his suspicion.

Sophia's husband offered to get his kidneys tested for a match in case a transplant was needed, but the doctor simply smiled and said that it wouldn't be necessary. He wasn't concerned, but he wouldn't say why. What did the doctor know, Sophia's husband wondered, that he didn't? The doctor was more concerned about getting a urine sample since Sophia wasn't producing any urine. After catheterizing Sophia, nurses were able to get enough urine for a lab test. A rush test revealed what the doctor had suspected all along. With the look of a detective who has just solved a crime, he explained that Sophia's state of shock had resulted from a basic urinary tract infection, which is fairly common among women. She probably hadn't felt anything when it started, but the infection had spread quickly upward and reached her kidney. It had entered her bloodstream, causing widespread activation of her immune system. Most likely it was the moment Sophia's immune system went into overdrive that she began to notice muscle tension.

The infection, the doctor explained, caused inflammation and irritation of the nerves in Sophia's left kidney and caused pain in the left side of her lower back. Her immune system was not able to control the infection, and she developed the overwhelming symptoms of exhaustion, weakness, fever, chills, nausea, and vomiting. These symptoms, when caused by infection, were collectively called sepsis. The individual symptoms could vary significantly, but the overwhelming sense of a body under stress was a telling symptom that Sophia should never have ignored. Without treatment, Sophia could have died.

But what about the kidney failure? Sophia's husband made his offer again. The doctor smiled and shook his head. There was no kidney failure, he explained. He couldn't have ruled it out completely before, but the tests had proved his suspicions correct: When Sophia's body went into shock from severe dehydration with sepsis, it triggered some mechanisms to try to conserve water. In the short term, the best way to conserve water is for the kidneys to shut down to prevent any water loss through urine. Sophia's blood pressure was so low that it could not sustain any more loss of water, so her kidneys stopped making urine and helped preserve water. Sophia was lucky—the loss of blood supply to the kidneys could have caused actual kidney damage if the interruption in blood flow had gone on long enough. It was a good thing she finally admitted she wasn't feeling right.

Sophia was treated in the hospital for four days with intravenous fluids and antibiotics. By the second day of treatment, her kidneys started to improve. She slowly regained her strength and even began walking around the hospital. Her appetite improved, and she began to eat and drink again. When her fever subsided, Sophia was discharged. She resumed work and felt like her old self again in every respect but one: she vowed to never ignore her body's signals ever again. She wasn't a burden to others when she was sick—she was no help to anyone if she could not help herself.

Teaching Points

Basic Approach: The Body Under Stress

No matter what the disease process is, your body has a certain way it reacts to dire physiological stress. It is important to recognize this reaction and seek help. To understand how to know when your body is in stress, you need to learn some basic physiological facts about bodily stress.

Like all animals, humans are programmed to respond to any threat with a fight-or-flight response. When animals sense any danger, they either prepare to fight the predator or to run away from it. The human body reacts in the same way when met with any type of threat. The threat may be outside the body or it may be internal. The greater the threat, the greater your body's response.

To understand how you react when your body is under stress due to a potentially life-threatening disease, you need to imagine how you might feel if you experienced a real life-threatening event. Imagine you are camping in a forest. Hiking through the woods, you disrupt a grizzly bear. The bear is frightened and appears ready to aggressively charge you. How does your body behave? Imagining this scenario, you may observe that your heart pounds in your chest, your pupils expand, and your palms begin to sweat. This type of stress response heightens your senses and prepares your body to face the threat. Now the grizzly turns around and goes back into the forest to mind its own business. You return to your camp. Your heart rate slowly goes down.

Your body exhibits a similar response when you have a rapidly progressing, possibly life-threatening disease brewing in your body. However, this type of physiological response is very taxing to the body. It takes a lot of energy to sustain the flight-or-flight response for a long time. When an illness is not cured, your body starts to lose the fight and crashes when it can no longer sustain fight-or-flight mode.

It is important to recognize when your body is going through this fight-or-flight crash phase. When you feel so sick that your body is unable to fight anymore, you are going through the fight-or-flight crash phase. If you do not seek help, the end result may be physiological shock, just like in Sophia's case. Your body will no longer be able to sustain the pounding of your heart, the increased muscle tension, and the high metabolism. When it gives up, your blood pressure will go down, and you will collapse.

Organ System: Renal

Renal failure and kidney infection were discussed in Sophia's story. Read on to learn the basics of the renal system and understand its role in health and sickness.

Your body can be viewed as a complex chemical factory. It uses food and oxygen to generate energy. It uses that energy to produce and sustain many different complex compounds that have unique functions in your body. Besides carbon and oxygen, nitrogen is the most commonly used element in these chemical processes. Your body mainly gets nitrogen from the protein you eat. Many by-products are formed during your body's essential chemical reactions. The main by-product is carbon dioxide, which is disposed of during the act of breathing. Other by-products consist of several chemicals containing the element nitrogen. These nitrogenous waste products are mainly eliminated by your kidneys.

You have two kidneys. Each kidney is packed with millions of "microfilters." Blood goes into each kidney from the big renal artery. This large blood vessel then divides into millions of small branches, each of which supplies blood to each microfilter. The blood is filtered and reabsorbed. The nitrogenous waste and other toxins remain in the filter and collect into small tubes that eventually merge and come out of each kidney as a single large tube. Two such tubes from the two kidneys drain into the urinary bladder. The filtered substance produced is urine. It gets rid of waste by-products for your kidneys.

Because of the sophisticated structure of the kidneys, they can influence your body function in more ways than just by filtering your blood. One very important function of the kidneys is to regulate the volume of the blood circulating in your body. Blood is 60 percent water. The volume of blood depends on the volume of water circulating in your blood vessels. Kidneys have a very elaborate mechanism to control the amount of water in your blood. They basically make more urine if there is too much water in the blood. They make less urine if there is not enough circulating blood volume. The kidneys control the amount of urine by controlling the amount of water reabsorbed from the urine and the amount of blood filtered.

We estimate kidney function by measuring the amount of nitrogenous waste in blood. If the amount is low enough, we infer that the kidneys are doing a good job eliminating the waste. If the amount is high, we infer that the kidney function has declined because they have not been effective in clearing out these compounds. The level of these compounds can be used to estimate kidney function. In people who have complete kidney failure, all the microfilters are clogged or damaged. They can no longer filter blood and make urine.

All our body's organs have a natural tendency to do what they can to fight immediate, life-threatening problems. These short-term strategies are in sync with the fight-or-flight approach. They prepare you for the immediate danger, but they cannot sustain you for long. Kidneys are no exception. When your kidneys sense that there is an immediate danger of shock due to lack of circulating blood, the priority is maintaining blood volume at all costs. In such a dire situation, the kidneys slow down or completely shut off the production of urine to preserve blood volume. As a result, toxic waste starts to accumulate. In the short term, the amount of toxic waste accumulated over a few hours won't kill you, but collapsed blood circulation might.

In cases of shock, such as Sophia's, kidney shutdown can be treated if the shock is reversed quickly enough. However, it can result in actual kidney failure if you wait too long. When kidneys shut down the production of urine, they do so by decreasing the amount of blood that reaches the microfilters and their tiny blood vessels. If the blood supply is interrupted for too long, these delicate units begin to die off because of the lack of enough oxygen and nutrients. When kidneys stop making urine, it is a dire signal that the body is fighting for survival. As doctors treat a person with shock, the kidneys start to recover and make urine again. Inadequate urine output is a sign that a particular treatment is ineffective; that's why very sick patients in the ICU have dedicated staff and equipment to measure the exact amount of urine they are making at all times. In this particular case, our patient had reversible kidney failure. There are many other causes of kidney failure that are not this instantaneously dramatic but rather happen over a long period of time. Many such kidney failures are not reversible. In those cases, there is no dramatic change in blood volume, but toxins start to accumulate. Those patients may not have any symptoms for many years until the majority of the filtering units have been damaged. Their symptoms appear when the toxin level is so high that it interferes with normal bodily functions.

3. Listen to Your Heart

How Mark's Intuition Saved His Life

Being vigilant about the possibility of a heart attack, no matter what symptoms you have, can be more important than whether your symptoms point to a heart attack.

The morning after Christmas, Mark woke up around nine and looked out the window to see more than a foot of snow covering his driveway. Steeling himself, he got dressed and went down to the garage to take a closer look at the snow before getting ready for the task that lay ahead of him—clearing the driveway.

Mark's wife and kids were still sleeping off the excitement of the day before. After a quick cup of coffee, Mark went back to his garage and pulled out the snow blower. After a good fifteen minutes of revving the machine's engine to no effect, Mark realized he'd have to clear the driveway the old-fashioned way.

After about five minutes of shoveling, Mark noticed some unusual heaviness in his left arm. He was left handed, so he decided to take a break, after which he resumed his shoveling. Ten minutes later, the heavy sensation returned, this time bringing with it some shoulder pain, as though he'd pulled a muscle in his left arm. Despite the pain and discomfort, Mark pushed on for another ten minutes, taking it a bit slower. He still had half the driveway to clear. The pain eased off as he slowed down, and he allowed himself to take another twenty minutes to clear the driveway instead of rushing through the job. Afterward he came back inside and sat down. There was still some residual soreness in his arm, so he stretched his shoulder a bit. At first, this seemed to help. Eventually, however, the soreness returned.

When Mark came back inside, his wife and kids were making breakfast in the kitchen. As soon as his wife saw him, she was worried—he looked pale and exhausted. Even sitting down in the warm kitchen, his pain eased off, but the dull ache never went away. When the pain persisted for another thirty minutes, Mark's wife called their doctor's office. There was no answer at the office the day after Christmas, but Mark's wife left a message and got a call back right away from a nurse. The nurse asked if moving Mark's shoulder made the pain any worse. He explained that it did and that while the soreness subsided when he slowed down, the ache never went away. Assuming Mark had pulled a muscle shoveling the driveway, the nurse told Mark to take some Tylenol and to get some rest.

Mark didn't need to be told twice. He was so exhausted that he didn't even have the energy to eat breakfast. His appetite was also gone, and the smell of food made him feel sick. This weakness made Mark think. He hadn't been sick in a long time, and he'd never felt like this before. He was normally very active and conscientious about his health. He would never think of himself as the kind of person who would be done in by thirty minutes of shoveling snow. He realized something must really be wrong, and despite the nurse's diagnosis of a pulled muscle, he told his wife something just didn't feel right. She drove him to the ER immediately.

The ER was extremely busy the day after Christmas; accidents were frequent during the holiday season. Mark spoke briefly to the registration nurse, explaining his activity prior to his symptoms, shoveling snow, and describing his most concrete symptoms, the pain and pressure in his shoulder, in detail. The nurse checked his vitals and wrote down "shoulder pain after shoveling snow" as his primary complaint.

Mark sat down to wait. The aching in his shoulder continued, and he felt weaker. His nausea was getting worse as well, but he didn't want to say anything. He could wait. There were so many other sick and injured people waiting in the ER who probably needed more urgent attention. He didn't want to overreact or be a nuisance since he'd gotten a diagnosis. He waited patiently for more than twenty minutes and all the while the ache in his shoulder continued. He felt weaker, and his nausea worsened, but he also felt silly asking for help when he'd already been told he had probably just pulled a muscle. But when Mark started to feel so sick that he could hardly sit up, he knew there was something seriously wrong. He needed immediate help. His wife went over to the nursing desk and asked for help. The nurse checked his vitals and put him on stretcher. Mark was wheeled off to a private room. The nurse called the ER doctor and received an order for a stat (rush) EKG. The doctor, she explained, wanted to do a rapid heart attack assessment.

Without delay, Mark was hooked up to a heart monitor, and blood tests and oxygen were administered. The first test came back in twenty minutes, and the result was clear: critical. Mark's troponin level was twenty milligrams per deciliter (mg/dl). Troponin is a special enzyme specific to heart muscles. When there is any damage to the heart muscle cells, these enzymes are released into the blood. Normally the level of troponin in the blood is very low—less than 0.04 mg/dl. The exact level depends on the particular lab and the specific method they use to test it. Sometimes values up to 0.9 may be considered normal, but anything above 0.9 is high. A high troponin level is indicative of damage to the heart muscles. The higher the troponin level, the more serious the damage.

Injury and breakdown of heart muscles can result from a number of different causes, but a heart attack is the most common cause of heart muscle injury. In most cases, an elevated troponin level usually points to the occurrence of a heart attack. Knowing this, the ER doctor asked Mark to tell him exactly what had happened when the symptoms began. He needed to find out if Mark's story matched up with the lab findings. Mark's story checked out—when he exerted himself in the cold weather by trying to shovel snow too quickly, he had a heart attack. One of the arteries supplying blood to his heart muscles had most likely narrowed, and as he shoveled snow, the workload on his heart had increased significantly. At first, Mark had experienced discomfort in his arm as the narrow artery was not able to supply enough blood to meet the needs of his heart. As he rested, demand on his heart decreased temporarily, and his discomfort decreased accordingly. As he started working again, the blood supply to his heart was no longer sufficient, and that deficiency caused his shoulder pain. Eventually the lack of blood flow got so much worse that even when he decreased his activity, Mark's blood flow was still too low—his arteries were just too narrow. When the lack of blood supply stunned part of his heart, Mark began to have a heart attack. But if he had a heart attack, why did Mark's shoulder ache and not his chest?

The doctor knew that the wiring of the nerves connected to the body's heart muscles was very different from the wiring of nerves to the other muscles in the body. For example, the muscles in your arms are directly wired to your nerve tissue in a way that transmits any damage or pressure in your arm muscles directly to the brain without interference so that the brain immediately recognizes the pain or discomfort coming from that particular region of your arm. Your heart muscles are wired differently. If their movements were directly transmitted to the brain, you would feel your heart pounding all the time. To avoid this distraction, the nerves connected to your heart muscles wire information to the unconscious, automated part of the brain. These nerves carry indirect sensations of heart pain to the brain by associating them with other nerves that travel together, like the nerves attached to Mark's arm muscles. Although the exact pathways of nerve association can vary, most people feel heart damage in the middle of their chests. However, the pain may be felt in additional locations, such as the neck, jaw, shoulder, or even in the stomach.

Mark was rushed to the catheterization lab, a special operating room designed to treat patients like Mark, who came in with heart attacks or blocked arteries. He was sedated, and his groin was numbed so that a complex procedure could be performed. A thick needle was inserted into a large artery in his groin. A heart catheter (a tube with a special balloon tip) was passed into the artery and pushed all the way up to Mark's heart. The doctor injected a special dye into the catheter so that the blood vessels downstream from the catheter could be viewed on x-ray. He slowly advanced the catheter inside the heart and then into the artery that supplied blood to the heart muscle itself, where he found an almost complete blockage inside a left-sided branch of the artery. To open the blockage, he used the balloon at the tip of the catheter. After widening the blocked artery, he placed a small round piece of metal tube (a stent) inside and injected the dye again to make sure that blood was flowing normally to all parts of the heart. When he eventually saw that it was, he retracted the catheter and closed the entry point. After a short time in recovery, Mark was transported back to the cardiac floor.

When the sedation wore off, Mark found that his pain had disappeared. He felt much better. The doctor monitored Mark's heart rate all night and gave him medication intravenously to thin his blood and prevent any further clogging. The next morning, an ultrasound of Mark's heart showed that no permanent damage had been done to his heart muscles. The operation had restored blood flow to his heart before there could be any significant, long-lasting damage.

"Well," the doctor said, smiling, "it looks like you came to us in the nick of time. Be sure to take care of yourself in the new year."

"I'm glad too," Mark replied.

Teaching Points

Basic Approach: Listen to Your Heart

Even if you know and trust your doctor and assisting nurses, you can't always rely on them to know how you're feeling. Sometimes it's difficult to describe exactly how you feel, and it can be just as hard for a doctor to work with a patient's description of his or her symptoms. You can describe your symptoms as objectively as possible, and sometimes your symptoms may only be taken at face value, without an understanding of how you're feeling. Sometimes, like Mark, it's best to listen to your body and not to the initial diagnosis. Otherwise your diagnosis might be delayed or even incorrect. Mark told his doctor's nurse and the ER nurse everything he could. He even told them what kind of pain he was experiencing. He didn't tell them that the pain made him feel as though something was very wrong or that he'd never experienced that sort of pain before. Although initially hesitant to ask for another opinion or assistance, Mark finally listened to his body and realized he needed urgent care. His intuition was fortunate, as was his wife's determination to summon the nurse in a very crowded ER on the day after Christmas. Had they waited another hour, Mark could have died.

When you have a major catastrophe in your body, your body sends you an SOS. Since everyone's body reacts differently, it's often hard to pinpoint or label the exact signal your body is sending. For some people, that signal feels like, "I'm going to die." For others, it may feel like, "My body is drained of energy," or simply, "Something is seriously wrong." Don't take a symptom at face value and search for a disease or condition to match. Take into consideration how that symptom makes you feel.

Organ System: The Heart

The heart is the most important organ in the body. In order to understand what a heart attack is, you need to know a little more about your heart's structure and function. Even before you read chapter 2, you probably knew that the heart pumped blood. It has two sides—the left and the right. Each side has an upper chamber and a lower chamber. The upper chambers mainly collect blood and push it down to the lower chambers. The lower chambers pump the blood out. The right side pumps the blood into your lungs, where the blood gets its oxygen supply. It then returns to the left side. The left side pumps this oxygenated blood to the rest of the body. The used-up blood finally returns to the right side to be pumped back into your lungs again. No part of your body can survive without a constant supply of the freshly oxygenated blood—not even the heart itself.

The heart has strong muscles that contract to supply the force needed to pump blood to your body. These muscles need a supply of fresh blood with oxygen and nutrients to churn out the energy the heart needs to keep functioning. These heart muscles cannot use the blood that is inside the heart because the blood needs to go deep inside the muscles to be able to feed the energy generating cells living inside. To supply blood to those muscle cells, the heart connects directly to two arteries that repenetrate the heart muscles and then branch off to supply blood to all the muscle cells in the heart walls. These arteries are called coronary arteries—the same arteries that, when blocked, cause heart attacks. When a branch of the coronary artery gets blocked, a part of the heart does not receive oxygen and nutrition. This deficiency causes you to have a heart attack.

When the blood supply is reduced but not cut off, the artery is sometimes narrowed but not completely blocked. Your heart muscles exhibit signs of being under stress. You experience pain when your heart needs to work a little harder. You may have pain when you walk or run, but you shouldn't have it at rest as Mark did. Heart pain when you walk or run is stable angina. Heart pain when you are at rest is called unstable angina. Angina may be the harbinger of a heart attack. Fortunately it takes a while for your heart muscles to die after the blood supply is cut off. If you seek treatment right away and get the correct diagnosis, like Mark eventually did, a doctor can restore your blood supply and save your heart muscles.

At this point in the chapter, you may be tempted to look up "symptoms of a heart attack" or "symptoms of angina" so that you can recognize the signs in case you or a loved one experiences angina. However, the list of symptoms associated with angina or a heart attack may not match your symptoms. Instead of memorizing the list of common symptoms associated with angina or a heart attack, it's far more important to know how you may feel and why you may feel that way.

When the supply of blood to an area of your heart is reduced or blocked, that part of the heart goes into severe distress due to lack of oxygen. This deficiency alters the muscles' metabolism and forces your muscles to leak enzymes and function improperly. The distress signals your muscles send out travel through nerves and reach your brain. As Mark's doctor knew earlier, however, your brain doesn't hear the distress signal from your heart as it would any other distress signal.

When you prick your finger, you immediately experience pain in that finger since your finger has very sensitive nerves that carry the pain signal directly and unequivocally to your brain. Your brain can identify and pinpoint the location of your finger's pain. Your heart does not have any such nerve. Most of the nerve fiber that your heart gets belongs to the autonomic nervous system that does not register pain. Nerves connected to your heart muscles only transport data to and from the brain that are necessary to regulate your heartbeat, a task that is carried out autonomously without your knowledge. When you have a heart attack, you only feel the accompanying pain because the nerves from your heart travel through and merge with other nerves that transmit pain from other body parts. These body parts may include your chest wall, your arms, your shoulders, your neck, your jaw, and surrounding areas. The exact pattern and path of the nerves may be slightly variable in different people.

Although you may not feel direct pain when you have a heart attack, it's important to pay attention to how you feel because your heart muscles send data to your brain that contains a distress signal, interpreted by your brain as pain from other parts of your body. That is why pain from a heart attack or angina can often seem very vague. It may not even feel like pain at all. It may just feel like pressure, discomfort, or some kind of ache; it may even manifest simply as nausea. Whenever you feel any of these sensations in the appropriate setting, you need to make sure you are not having a heart attack. The best way to do that is to go to the nearest ER and tell them that you are worried about a possible heart attack.

4. Drowned Out

*How the Sensation of Drowning Was Really an SOS
from Anita's Body*

*What you feel is what your body is trying to tell you.
This principle will help you understand the mechanism
of the heart as well as the symptoms of congestive heart
failure.*

Anita woke up in the night gasping for air. She was
sitting in her own bed, but her body felt like it was
drowning in a lake, like her head was underwater. She
sat up straight, as if she was trying to keep her head
above water. To her surprise, the technique actually
worked. Her breathing improved as she propped her
head up, but now she started to get a bit scared. She lay
back down to try to fall asleep—and it happened again.
That same feeling of being underwater came back. Now
this was terrifying. What was happening? Lately Anita
hadn't felt like herself. She'd been having trouble
sleeping, which was unusual. Usually she felt like she
slept too much, but lately she had felt uncomfortable in
her own bed. It seemed like something was blocking her
air passage whenever she lay down. She had to sit up to
get more air, but tonight was new. Anita got out of the
bed, stood up, and decided to call her doctor.

Anita knew she was not in great shape, but in the past
month, things seemed to be getting worse. A longtime
diabetic, she struggled to keep her blood sugar at the
level recommended by her doctor. She took medication
for her high blood pressure and cholesterol problems,
but her biggest health problem was her weight. She had
tried dozens of different diet techniques but had never
been able to significantly lose weight—her knees were
bad, and they made exercise difficult.

Every time Anita tried to exercise, her knees gave out under the pressure. She didn't know anymore which problem had started first. Despite all these troubles, she did what she could to improve her health. She watched what she ate, took water aerobics classes twice a week, took her pills on time, gave up smoking, and did not miss her doctor's appointments. It was a struggle, but she was taking steps in the right direction.

She always felt tired because she was overweight. At five and a half feet tall and three hundred and forty pounds, she was medically classified as obese. Walking was often difficult, and she always walked slowly, watching her steps, to avoid falling. Since she moved slowly and carefully, it took Anita a few weeks to notice that she was running out of breath more and more easily. She used to be able to walk up and down the stairs in her house fairly easily, stopping only to rest her knees but never to catch her breath. In the last few weeks, however, she noticed that just a flight of stairs could easily wind her. Soon just walking down the hallway became a struggle. In the past few days, things had looked even worse. She would become breathless just after walking a few steps. That was when she started having trouble sleeping. And now here she was, gasping for air in her own bed. Anita dialed her doctor's number anxiously. She wasn't sure she'd live through another episode like the one she'd just had, and she didn't want to find out.

Luckily Anita had a wonderful family doctor who knew her very well. The nurse picked up the phone and, sensing the urgency in Anita's voice, fetched the doctor immediately. Anita told her doctor exactly how she had felt in the last few weeks and explained what was happening to her in the last few days. The doctor listened to her very attentively, without interrupting, and asked her a few more questions after she was finished. She could hear the concern in his voice.

"Anita," her doctor said, "I just want you to stay right where you are and to stay calm. We need to get you down to the ER as soon as possible—this sounds like a heart problem. But I don't want you to worry. We'll make all the arrangements for you since we have your home address here. You just stay there and wait for the ambulance. Can you do that for me?"

Anita confessed that she was very scared, but she thought she could wait. Her doctor thanked her. He could only imagine how alarmed she must be, but he knew Anita was in danger and that whatever heart problem she was having needed to be solved as soon as possible. He told her to remain calm and to call back if the ambulance didn't arrive in fifteen minutes. Anita waited quietly, but she was anxious. When the paramedics arrived to take her vitals and transport her to the ER, they put her on oxygen and called the ER nurse to prepare her for Anita's arrival. All this frightened Anita even more.

"Will I be OK?" she asked them.

"Your oxygen is a bit low, but your other vitals are OK," one paramedic told her. She shouldn't worry, though, because the doctor would see her as soon as she got to the ER, he explained. Anita felt a little better, but not much.

As soon as the ambulance reached the ER, a nurse rushed out to direct the paramedics to the room that had been prepared for Anita. She was transferred from a stretcher to the bed fairly quickly, and Anita was relieved to find that in bed, she could prop her head up higher to get more air. The oxygen helped, but she still needed to keep her head up above the invisible water to breathe. She was so exhausted by the effort that she felt she wouldn't be able to keep herself afloat much longer.

The water felt like it was getting higher, but she could only raise her head up so far. The nurse propped the bed up as high as it would go. Sitting almost straight up, Anita felt like she could finally take deeper breaths.

The ER doctor rushed in as soon as Anita was settled in. He asked her a few questions. She told him how she had been feeling the last few weeks and how breathing had become more difficult, even over the last few days. It was a struggle even to speak the words, but she managed to finish her story. After a quick examination, the doctor spoke.

"Anita, I am worried about the condition of your heart," he said. "It seems like your heart is not pumping enough blood out of your lungs. I want to run a few tests to confirm the diagnosis. As soon as I have some preliminary results, I can start treatment, and we can get you on the road to feeling a bit better. But first, we'll need to do a quick x-ray."

He motioned to the radiology technician waiting outside with a portable x-ray machine and stepped outside. After the x-ray scans were complete, he stepped back in to examine the resulting images of Anita's chest.

"No wonder you feel like you're drowning," he said, shaking his head. "Your lungs are filled with liquid, and your heart appears to be enlarged. Most likely you're having heart failure. I still need to do some more tests to be sure, but there's no time to waste so I will be starting you on some medications as soon as you're hooked up to an IV. Don't worry I'll be back to explain shortly."

As the doctor exited, a nurse entered with a syringe and a few test tubes. First she drew some blood and then inserted and secured an IV line into Anita's vein. She hooked up another syringe—this one filled with fluid.

"The doctor has ordered some IV Lasix for you," she explained. "Lasix will help get rid of that extra fluid in your lungs. Now I'll also need to insert a urinary catheter to measure how much urine came out as a result of that medicine. Do you think you can be a bit brave for me? I know this must all be frightening." Anita nodded. The procedure sounded very uncomfortable, but she knew it was necessary. The urinary catheter was secured in place, and her urine was draining into a plastic bag with measuring labels. The nurse moved Anita up to the cardiac floor and kept the heart monitor and oxygen on all night. Anita was given medication to enhance urine production, and it helped her heal by leaps and bounds. Her breathing improved overnight as she got rid of a large amount of water through her urine.

The next morning, an echocardiogram of Anita's heart showed that her heart muscles were, in fact, working very poorly—her heart was only pumping out about 30 percent of the blood that it received. After two days of hospitalization, however, Anita's breathing improved significantly. After making a follow-up appointment with a heart specialist and getting further preventative information on heart failure, Anita was discharged on oxygen. She was finally going home.

Teaching Points

Basic Approach: Shortness of Breath

Your body always tries to tell you when something is wrong. That's why it's so important to listen carefully to your body and verbalize exactly what you're experiencing. In addition to describing your symptoms, describe what they feel like. If it feels like you are being choked, say you feel like you are being choked. If it feels like you are drowning, say you feel like you are drowning. When you clearly say what you think is happening to your body, you quickly direct the attention of your doctor to the correct disease process. It will expedite your diagnosis and treatment.

Shortness of breath after heavy exercise is normal. But if walking winds you, shortness of breath may be a sign of a serious problem. The mechanics of breathing in and out are controlled by multiple organ systems—your heart, your lungs, or your blood system—any of whose dysfunction can cause shortness of breath. That's why any small detail about how you feel when you experience breathlessness can be a significant step toward a proper diagnosis.

Organ System: The Pumping Heart

In the previous chapter on heart attack, you learned how blood is supplied to the heart muscles. Having read Anita's story, you've now seen that the heart performs many functions. As you now know, your heart has a right side and a left side. The right side pumps blood to your lungs, which, in turn, oxygenate the blood and return it to the left side. The left side then pumps blood out to the rest of the body, excluding the lungs. Used blood from your body returns to the right side to be pumped back to the lungs again. This whole process is known as a cardiac cycle, which is made up of two phases: contraction and relaxation. During the contraction phase, heart muscles contract and pump blood out. During the relaxation phase, the heart muscles relax and collect returning blood.

Heart failure sets in when the heart begins less effectively pumping blood and can arise because of a malfunction during either the contraction or relaxation phase. Symptoms of problems in either phase are often identical, so observing symptoms may not always be the best way to determine the origin of the failure.

Sometimes the word "failure" can be confusing; it sounds like all heart failure occurs suddenly, causing an instant collapse or death. Sudden collapse and death resulting from cardiac problems, however, are referred to

45

as "sudden cardiac death" and may not be related to pump failure. Most heart failure occurs over months and years—you may go a long period of time without feeling any specific symptoms from your heart failure. Since heart failure happens slowly, your body adapts to the inefficient pumping. While your body's ability to adapt to heart failure is beneficial in the short run, it causes most heart problems in the long term since symptoms emerge only when the adaptive mechanism is no longer able to sustain near-normal functioning.

When your heart begins to pump blood inefficiently to your body, blood flow starts to lag. Blood flowing from the lungs to the left side of the heart becomes congested, increasing pressure inside the blood vessels in the lungs. This increased pressure causes your lungs to swell and accumulate fluid. Wet and swollen, your lungs struggle to absorb enough oxygen, and you feel very short of breath. Like Anita, your shortness of breath gets worse when you lie down because more fluid backs up into your lungs in that position.

Heart failure is sometimes caused by issues that can be corrected, such as by leaking heart valves or oxygen-deprived heart muscles. If the heart failure is indeed caused by one of these problems, treatment specific to the cause may be necessary. Otherwise treatment for heart failure includes medication and lifestyle changes. Most of the medicines are used to counteract your body's natural adaptive mechanism in heart failure. They prevent modification of your heart muscles and blood vessels that will avoid or delay chronic health problems caused by heart failure. In the meantime, careful adjustment and fine tuning of the amount of salt and water in the body, with low-salt diet and diuretics, will help with lung swelling and fluid accumulation as well as aid in improving your breathing. Either way, whether medication or more specialized treatment is necessary, it's extremely important to seek help immediately for heart problems. The longer you wait, the less your chance of recovery.

The actual treatment guidelines for heart failure have recently been the topic of fruitful research, with many new and promising treatment regimens being tested every year. You can read the latest news and expert advice on the topic on the American Heart Association's (AHA) website.

5. Body, Meet Brain

How Falling Unconscious Raised Emily's Consciousness

Even an unconscious person has a story to tell. Although your brain controls your state of consciousness, unconsciousness is not always caused by a problem in the brain.

The night Emily had a seizure, the whole family was over at her country home for dinner—her daughter, son-in-law, and her grandkids. Dinner was ready, and her daughter had just finished setting the table. Emily had gone to wash her hands, but when she came back from the bathroom, her daughter noticed that she looked pale and exhausted. She closed her eyes slowly, as if about to faint. As her daughter ran toward her, Emily slumped over, falling to the ground. Her daughter expected her to be limp, but her body became incredibly stiff, and her arms and legs began to shake in what seemed like rhythmic contraction, as if responding to a dream. Her family looked on in horror as Emily shook, making loud, senseless noises. Her daughter called 911 and described her mother's state over the phone. All of a sudden, Emily stopped moving, as though she had fallen into a deep sleep on the floor, with her face displaying no pain, and her breaths coming quick and shallow. When her daughter tried to wake her, she didn't respond. The ambulance arrived in five minutes. The paramedics immediately put an oxygen tube in Emily's mouth, listened to her heart, and checked her blood pressure. Placing her on a stretcher, they wheeled her out to an ambulance. Once inside, they stuck a wire to Emily's chest and performed an EKG (electrocardiogram) test, electronically transmitting the EKG data to the nearest ER in the rural area.

That winter, Emily had just turned seventy-two. Although she had always been relatively healthy, she was a heavy, pack-a-day smoker. Aside from a "smoker's cough" in the morning, though, she rarely had any health problems. But over the last few weeks, she had been feeling tired, and walking, her favorite form of exercise, had begun to wind her. All this she had regarded as the price of getting older.

When the ambulance arrived at the nearest ER, Emily was still unconscious. A nurse checked her vitals and observed that she looked all right—no fever, normal blood pressure, and heart rate and rhythm. Because of the oxygen tube, she was breathing normally, at a low flow setting of two liters per minute. She performed a follow-up EKG and took some blood for tests. An ER doctor reviewed the EKGs and blood tests but was unable to find anything that might explain Emily's symptoms. Taking her daughter aside, he discussed Emily's condition.

"Emily has had a seizure, but we don't yet know what caused it. I'm a bit concerned about the fact that she's still unresponsive, so I think it might be better to move her to the nearest city hospital, where they can run more tests and get some specialists to see her."

The daughter agreed, and the hospital made arrangements for Emily's transfer. An hour later, she was lying in the intensive care unit at the city hospital—a much larger institution. As a new doctor examined her, he attempted to wake her. Emily slept on. Turning to Emily's daughter, the doctor asked whether she had been present when her mother had become unresponsive.

Emily's daughter nodded. "Yes, my husband and kids were there as well. She'd just gone to wash her hands."

"Well, I'm very glad you were there. If you can, please walk me through what happened in as much detail as you can. I know this must be very upsetting, but what you tell me may save your mother's life since she can't tell me herself." Emily's daughter nodded again, fiercely blinking back tears. She described every detail as vividly as she could. Glancing at Emily's chart, the doctor stopped her. "I'm just going to interrupt for a moment—your mother's chart says she is a smoker. Can you talk to me about that?"

Emily's daughter nodded again. "She's been smoking since she was a teenager. She did try to cut down a few years back, but now she's back up to a pack a day again. It gives her a pretty nasty cough in the morning, but otherwise she's seemed fine."

"Are you sure?" the doctor asked.

"Well," the daughter said slowly, "my mother hasn't been to see a doctor in years. I guess we don't really know if she's had other problems related to her smoking."

"That's all right," the doctor assured her. "You're being very helpful. Have you noticed any change in her health in the last few years?"

Emily shook her head. Her mother only ever complained that she was getting older. The doctor pressed further, saying, "Did she mention anything specific that was bothering her?"

"Walking," Emily remembered. "Lately she's been saying she doesn't have all the energy she used to have. She loves walking and jogging. She used to walk for miles without getting tired. Now she has to slow down to catch her breath. That's why she tried to cut back on smoking, you see, but she just couldn't seem to quit."

The doctor ordered some blood work and a chest x-ray as well as a CAT scan of Emily's head. Within thirty minutes, the results were back. The CT scan of her head appeared normal, but the chest x-ray showed abnormalities. Years of heavy smoking had taken a toll on Emily's lungs. Stiff and sluggish, her lungs didn't appear to be recoiling to the normal position at the end of a breath. They were abnormal in shape and size as well—unusually large and barrel shaped.

After looking at the chest x-ray, the doctor took Emily's daughter aside again. He suspected Emily had COPD, a disease of the lungs that occurs in people who smoke cigarettes.

The daughter looked at him, confused. "But what does that have to do with my mother not waking up?"

"I'm waiting for a blood-gas analysis, which should confirm a connection between your mother's smoking and her current unconscious state. A blood-gas analysis is a special blood test that takes blood out of an artery in the wrist and analyzes it for oxygen and carbon dioxide.

"But didn't the nurse just say her breathing was OK?" Emily's daughter asked. "Her oxygen level was more than ninety-five percent—isn't that good enough?"

"Yes and no," the doctor said. "You see, the nurse can estimate the amount of oxygen in your mother's blood with a finger clip, but she can't estimate the amount of carbon dioxide in the blood with it. We need to actually analyze the blood inside her artery to measure its carbon-dioxide content. Sometimes abnormal carbon dioxide can cause confusion and unresponsiveness. In extreme conditions, it can trigger a seizure."

A specially trained lab technician came to Emily's bedside and started checking for her pulse in her left wrist. He took his time feeling the pulse before he took out his blood-gas syringe. He punctured Emily's skin right at the spot where he had felt the strongest pulse, and the needle went straight inside the artery that was pulsating with freshly oxygenated blood. The doctor explained that it took special training and experience to be able to stick the needle directly inside an artery to draw an arterial blood sample. While it was relatively easy to draw blood from veins because they ran near the skin's surface and were visible and recognizable by their bluish hue, it was much more difficult to draw blood from arteries because they couldn't be seen directly. The position of arteries could only be estimated by feeling the high pulse created by the high pressure of these blood vessels, as the lab technician did.

The reason that two different systems of blood vessels existed, he continued, was that the two systems carried blood in two states of oxygenation to the body. The arterial system carried freshly oxygenated blood, and the venous system carried used-up blood that lacked oxygen. The arterial system was made up of thick-walled, pulsating blood vessels that carried the high-oxygen, high-pressure blood from the heart to every single cell in the body. The oxygen in this blood was what kept the cells in every organ alive. When the organs used up all the oxygen in the blood, they produced carbon dioxide as a waste product that needed to be disposed of. That's where the system of blood vessels known as the venous system came in—taking the used blood, along with the carbon dioxide, back to the heart for processing via low pressure. The venous system had lower pressure than the arterial system because the walls of the venous system blood vessels were much thinner than those in the arterial system, since used blood had much lower pressure than freshly pumped blood. The blood flowing inside the veins appeared bluish in color due to the lack of oxygen. The fresh blood running at high pressure inside the arteries had a bright-red color.

To analyze the accurate amount of oxygen and carbon dioxide in the blood, the doctor needed a blood sample from Emily's artery. The doctor asked the technician to run the sample analysis at a bedside mobile blood analyzer—sending it to the lab could take time Emily didn't have.

Within a few seconds, the doctor had the answer. The CO_2 level in Emily's blood was 110, the highest the doctor had ever seen. The normal level was around forty. A level as high as Emily's could affect the brain and could certainly lead directly to a seizure and general unresponsiveness.

When he explained this to Emily's daughter, she was very worried. "Will she ever wake up?" she asked.

"Well, we do have ways to bring the CO_2 down," the doctor said hesitantly. "That is what I want to talk to you about. We have two possible ways of bringing down her CO_2 levels at this time. The first option is to put a tube down her throat, connect the tube to a ventilator, and have the machine blow off the extra CO_2 out from her lungs. It's the most reliable option, as the ventilator gives us a very controlled environment. But the problem with this approach is that intubating is very invasive. Your mother will be very uncomfortable and will need narcotics and sedatives to tolerate the ventilator. The other option is less invasive, but it doesn't always produce results. It is called BiPAP, bilevel positive airway pressure. We place a tight-fitting mask around her mouth and nose and then connect that mask to a machine. We use that machine to blow air in and out of her lungs. It's less reliable than the ventilator, but it is also less invasive. I think we should give the BiPAP a chance first. We can wait for three to four hours with the BiPAP and see how it works. If your mother's condition doesn't improve in the next four hours, we will have to intubate her and use the ventilator."

Emily's daughter agreed, and the doctor ordered the mask. The respiratory therapist came in and fit the mask tightly around Emily's mouth and nose and then connected it to the machine. It started blowing air into her lungs. They could see her chest rise with each blow.

The therapist was happy with the way the setup was working. In the next twenty minutes, Emily was moved up to a hospital bed in the ICU upstairs. The ER doctor handed over the case to the admitting doctor, who would take over Emily's care in the ICU. She was kept on the mask continually for about three hours before she began moving, appearing uncomfortable and attempting to remove the mask. A nurse called the doctor immediately. The doctor ordered another blood-gas analysis and reviewed the results, which were positive. Emily's CO2 levels had gone down to seventy-five. He ordered the respiratory therapist to temporarily remove the mask to see if Emily was awake. As soon as the mask was off, Emily woke up in a panic. She had no idea where she was.

The doctor introduced himself, relieved to finally be speaking to Emily. After explaining what had happened to her, he asked the question he had been hoping to ask since she came into the ER: "What was the last thing you remember before you lost consciousness?"

"I didn't know I lost consciousness, but I guess I did," Emily said. Shaking her head, she continued slowly. "I was feeling very tired, and my body felt a bit numb. I didn't want to say anything because I had family over for dinner. I didn't want to bother them. I hadn't slept well the night before and thought that I would feel better if I could just go to bed a bit early that night."

The doctor explained how Emily's CO2 level was sky-high. She would need to keep that mask on for at least another twelve hours before she would be out of danger.

Emily bravely tolerated the mask for another twelve hours. Her blood-gas level improved significantly. She was given inhalers, nicotine patches, and a follow-up appointment with a lung specialist. As her daughter drove her home, Emily thought about how lucky she was to be alive. As she looked at her daughter beside her, she made the decision to stop smoking for good.

Teaching Points

Basic Approach: The Patient Cannot Speak

Usually when you go to the doctor, you tell him or her how you feel. As you saw in previous chapters, information provided by the patient was crucial to the doctor's diagnosis. But what about when you are not able to speak for yourself, like Emily?

In such situations, your diagnosis is in the hands of your friends or your family. If your loved ones become sick in your presence and you are unable to communicate their symptoms or condition, their diagnoses, and possibly their lives, are in your hands. It's important to never assume that the doctor will reach the correct diagnosis on his or her own. Instead, always assume that the doctor will need to speak to someone, probably you, even though you aren't experiencing the symptoms, and you weren't necessarily present when the symptoms began. The information you have about the general health and habits of your loved ones may be extremely valuable in guiding the doctor in the right direction. Do not hold back information because it may be silly to mention. You never know what might help. Any change in daily routine, a new job, a change in medication, life stress, a recent trip, a change in mood or behavior, bad habits, addiction, or even hobbies may be the crucial information needed to lead the doctor to the right line of diagnostic thinking. These are just a few examples of things that might help, and there are definitely more. Just remember: You can never volunteer too much information when your ailing loved one is unable to speak.

Organ System: The Lungs

There are two important gas exchanges that occur in our lungs. Most of us know that we need oxygen to survive. We breathe in this oxygen from the air around us and then our lungs absorb it. As we take oxygen in, we blow carbon dioxide out. The exhalation of carbon dioxide is as important as the inhalation of oxygen itself. Too much CO_2 can be as bad as too little oxygen.

There are small air sacs inside our lungs, where the gas exchange takes place. All the air we breathe in eventually ends up inside these air sacs, which are the basic functional units in the lungs. The rest of each lung is made up of supporting tissue and blood vessels. The supporting tissue binds the blood vessels with the air sacs and maintains the structure of the lung.

Each air sac is supplied with tiny blood vessels with thin walls that allow the exchange of gases in and out of the blood. Gas from the air inside the air sac goes into the blood, and gas already in the blood goes out to the air, which then gets breathed out. Oxygen goes from air to blood because there is more oxygen in the air than in the blood inside the lungs. Carbon dioxide comes out from blood to air because there is more CO_2 in the blood than in the air. This difference in concentration is the driving force for the gas exchange, although the concentration of CO_2 varies much less than that of oxygen.

There are, however, differences in the way our lungs handle oxygen and CO_2. The exchange of CO_2 is much simpler than the exchange of oxygen because CO_2 diffuses more easily across the membrane of the air sacs.

When our breathing is not adequate, the gas inside the air sacs of the lungs do not easily mix with the atmospheric air, and the air we breathe in does not completely reach all the way to the air sacs. The air we breathe out does not completely empty the gases inside the air sacs to the outside air. When this movement of air in and out of the lungs is affected, you've got a ventilatory problem.

A ventilation problem causes a change in the concentration of oxygen and carbon dioxide inside the air sac of the lungs. As the concentration of CO_2 in the air sac goes up, the driving force of the gas exchange decreases, as the contrast in blood and air CO_2 levels grows less striking. As the exchange slows down, the concentration of CO_2 in the blood starts to rise. Since CO_2 levels contrast on a smaller scale than oxygen levels in the blood and the air, any change is felt more sharply. Oxygen exchange is usually more affected by problems related to the membrane than by problems in the ventilation system.

Emily had stiff lungs shaped like barrels that no longer expanded or contracted easily. They had lost their elasticity. When her lungs failed to expand and contract, her ventilation system stopped making the oxygen-CO_2 exchange. The exchange had been slowing down for many years, but the change was so slow that she did not notice it. Her body adapted to the higher level of CO_2 in the blood until it reached a critical point when her body could not tolerate it any longer. High CO_2 levels caused her brain to malfunction, which is why she had convulsions after her collapse and remained unresponsive until the doctors found a way to lower her CO_2 levels.

Not only can smoking make your lungs stiff, but they can also damage the lining or membrane of the air sacs inside the lungs. In some patients, only one type of damage is predominant. Patients who have more membrane damage present with problems of oxygen

57

exchange. Low oxygen makes them feel short of breath. Patients who have intact membranes with reduced ventilation may present with high CO_2 in the presence of near-normal oxygen. They may present in different ways depending on the extent and time course of the damage. In someone like Emily, who experienced many years of slow damage, symptoms may not appear until the body cannot survive anymore.

6. Confusion Solution

*How Kelly's Confusion Helped Clarify Her Diagnosis
for Her Doctor*

*Any change in the mental status in elderly patients can
be related to an underlying medical problem.*

At eighty-eight, Kelly was very healthy. A retired
attorney, she had three sons, one daughter, and twelve
grown grandchildren, all of whom regarded her as lively,
talkative, and mentally sharp. Her husband had passed
away two years ago, but her children and grandchildren
visited her regularly and loved talking to her. She always
had such interesting stories and touching memories to
share. This year, her children and their children got
together and threw a huge party for Kelly's birthday.
Kelly was touched to have such a loving family. Soon
the party would become another wonderful memory.

Shortly after Kelly's birthday, her oldest
granddaughter, Molly, noticed something very odd on a
visit to her grandmother's house. Kelly's house was a
mess. Usually Kelly kept the house very tidy, but this
day there were clothes on the floor and dirty dishes in
the sink.

"Are you all right, Grandma?" she asked. Kelly was
watching the news in her recliner, apparently
unperturbed by the mess around her.

"Oh, Molly, I'm so glad to see you!" Kelly said,
looking up. "I'm just fine. How have you been?"

"I'm fine too, Grandma…but are you sure you're all
right? It's a bit messy in here."

"Oh, sure, I'm absolutely fine. I just didn't get
around to finishing my laundry and dishes today. I'll do
them once I finish watching the news."

"Is there anything interesting on the news, Grandma?" Molly asked tentatively.

"Oh, yeah, there is this Supreme Court decision that I have been following. It takes me back to my days at the firm. But I don't want to bore you with the details."

"Well, why don't you enjoy watching the news while I finish up your dishes and put away your laundry?"

"Well, thanks, Molly. That's really kind of you." Kelly settled in once more.

After tidying up her grandmother's kitchen, Molly realized it was dinnertime. After ordering a pizza, she sat down to watch TV with her grandmother. When the pizza arrived, Molly noticed Kelly only had one slice. Her appetite was gone, she said, and she was tired. After tidying up a bit more, Molly left so that her grandmother could go to bed early. As she walked outside, she couldn't help feeling concerned. Her grandmother didn't usually accept help with work around the house. She always insisted on doing her chores herself. *Well, maybe something in the news spoiled her mood today*, Molly thought to herself as she drove home.

Still, the next morning, Molly wanted to check in on her grandmother one more time. After a quick breakfast, she drove to her grandmother's house. Kelly greeted her enthusiastically, but Molly realized something was wrong. It was nine in the morning on a Sunday, and her retired grandmother was wearing a business suit, as if she was going to work.

"Grandma, it's…awfully early to be dressed," Molly ventured. She didn't mention her grandmother's unusual choice of clothing.

"Well, it's time to go to work, Molly. I can't have my clients waiting for me. I'm so sorry but we'll have to chat another time—I'm running late."

"Grandma, what are you talking about?" Molly shook her head, baffled. Something wasn't right.

"Well, down at my law firm! I have a great assistant, of course, but there are some things only I can do. I'm so glad to see you, Molly, but I'd better get going."

Now Molly knew something was very wrong.

"Grandma! You have not been to the office in ten years! You sold the firm and retired ten years ago, remember?"

"What? What are you talking about?" Molly looked confused and suddenly very small in her pantsuit.

"Grandma," Molly said gently, "I think you aren't feeling well. Let me call your doctor right away. You don't work at the law firm anymore. Let me take care of you."

Molly called her father and her grandmother's doctor. The nurse at Kelly's doctor's office was concerned—she knew how sharp Kelly normally was. Such a dramatic change in Kelly's mental state overnight could mean Kelly needed immediate attention. She advised Molly to call 911.

Molly's father arrived at the same time as the paramedics to a very difficult scene. Kelly was upset and confused, still convinced she needed to go to work. As one of the paramedics tried to persuade her to get into the ambulance, Kelly waved his efforts off.

"You seem like a nice young man," she said. "My granddaughter is very stubborn, so would you please tell her that I'm fine so I can go to work? My clients are expecting me."

"I'm sure they are," the paramedic responded diplomatically, "but I think it's best to humor your granddaughter right now. Just let our ER doctor check you out first, and then we'll have you on your way." That seemed to do the trick.

At the nearest ER, the admitting nurse was glad they'd gotten Kelly to come in quickly. Kelly was weak and sweaty, and her heart rate was higher than normal—

115 beats per minute. Her blood pressure was slightly lower than normal as was her temperature.

"Can you tell me your full name?" the nurse asked.

Kelly nodded. "My name is Kelly Anderson."

"Kelly, do you know where you are?"

"Well, I was supposed to be at work," Kelly said pointedly, "but instead I'm in a hospital."

"Yes, Kelly. Do you know which hospital you're in?"

"Well, no. They didn't tell me which hospital they were taking me to."

"That makes sense," the nurse said reassuringly. "Do you know what day it is?"

"I don't know. No—wait—it must be Monday. I should be at work."

"Do you know what year it is?"

"Of course. It's 1996. Clinton just got reelected."

"I see," the nurse looked concerned. "I'll go find the doctor for you." She left the room hurriedly and returned with the ER doctor.

After a short conversation with Kelly, the doctor turned to Molly. "Can you tell me how your grandmother is when she is not sick?"

"Sorry, what do you mean? Is she sick?" Molly was worried.

"Does Kelly have trouble with her memory sometimes? She seems to think it's 1996, not 2014."

"No," Molly said, shaking her head. "She's always very sharp. You have to understand that this is not like Grandma at all. She's one of the smartest people I know. She was a very successful attorney before she retired."

"When was the last time you saw her before today?"

"I was at her house last night. We had pizza together."

"Was she acting normal last night?"

"Yes, she was still very sharp and smart. She was watching the news." Kelly paused and then added, "We even discussed current events. She knew what year it was."

"But was there anything different or unusual about her last night?" the doctor pressed.

Kelly thought for a moment. "Well, she did seem tired. She wanted to go to bed a little early."

"Did she complain of any pain, discomfort, or anything like that?"

"Nothing like that," Molly said. "Although now that you mention it, I was a little concerned. I don't know if I've ever seen her that tired. She's always so lively and active."

The doctor thanked Molly and ordered some blood tests and x-rays. He would come back, he told her, when the results started coming in. After a CT and a chest x-ray, technicians took Kelly's blood, and the nurse came back to start a saline solution IV. She handed Kelly a small plastic cup for a urine sample.

"Do I really need to do this?" Kelly protested. "I need to be at my law firm."

"Well," the nurse said patiently, "you're not well. The sooner you help us out, the sooner we can have you on your way to where you need to be."

"All right," Kelly said. "All right." The nurse followed Kelly into the bathroom. Kelly had trouble filling half the cup, and her urine appeared thick, cloudy, and pungent in smell.

Thirty minutes later, the doctor found Molly to show her some preliminary test results. Kelly's x-ray and her CAT scan were normal, but her blood tests were not. Her white blood-cell count was very high, her body was dehydrated, and her kidney function was slightly lower than normal. Overall her tests pointed to an overwhelming infection. Her chest x-ray showed no sign of infection in her lungs, but preliminary urine tests indicated a urine infection.

"She just has a urine infection?" Molly's dad asked. "I mean, are you sure? How can a urine infection cause such a dramatic change in a person? Shouldn't we be worried about a stroke?"

The doctor nodded. "Well, it's not uncommon for a urine infection to cause confusion and disorientation in people Kelly's age. So far, everything points to a urine infection. Her urine sample was loaded with white blood cells—the cells that fight infection and make pus. She doesn't have a fever, but her temperature is certainly lower than normal. At Kelly's age, a lower temperature is as significant as a higher temperature. Everything so far supports a severe UTI, including her confusion and disorientation."

"I'm sorry," Molly's father said, "but this is my mother. Is there any way to confirm this? I just don't want to take any chances. Could a UTI really cause all this?"

"Well, the only way to confirm your mother's condition is to start treatment and see whether she improves. If she doesn't start getting better in the next two to three days, we will start looking for other problems. At this point, I think we need to admit her to the hospital, watch her closely, and start treatment with antibiotics and IV fluids."

Kelly's son reluctantly conceded, and Kelly was transferred up to the medical floor, where the doctor started her on IV antibiotics and more IV fluids. Too tired to protest anymore, she simply closed her eyes and went to sleep. When she woke up the next morning, she felt better, like she was waking up from a strange dream she could only half remember. She knew she had been taken to the hospital, but she couldn't remember why, and she was still very weak and scared. She wanted to call the nurse and ask her what had happened to her, but she hesitated, embarrassed.

Once the nurse realized Kelly had woken up, she let Kelly's family into her room to see her.

"Grandma, how are you feeling now?" asked Molly.

"Well, sweetheart, I feel awfully tired and a little embarrassed," Kelly said. "Tell me what I did yesterday."

"You don't remember anything?" Molly frowned.

"I do remember, sort of. Like a bad dream," Kelly explained, "I remember bits and pieces, but I'm not sure if everything really happened or if I dreamed it."

"Apparently you had a bad infection, and it made you a little confused. You thought you were still working at the law firm. When we realized you weren't all right, we brought you here."

"No!" Kelly exclaimed, embarrassed. "Did I do anything too silly?"

"No," Molly said. She decided not to tell her mother about the pantsuit incident. "You just kept saying you needed to be at work. But, eventually, you let the nurses and doctors treat you. So how are you feeling?"

"Well, at least I've come to my senses now. I'm still very tired, but I don't hurt anywhere."

"Grandma, we're so glad," Molly said. "You may need another couple of days in the hospital, so just take it easy for a bit."

"Well," Kelly said, smiling weakly, "it's a good thing I don't have to go to work!"

Teaching Points

Basic Approach: Confusion

Confusion in an elderly person can be a very important diagnostic clue and should not be ignored. Your brain is the most important organ in your body. When there is a sudden change in the way your brain functions, it's a sign that your body is in grave danger.

Your body has evolved to protect your brain from danger at all cost. When your body encounters possibly life-threatening changes, it always tries to protect your brain. For example, when you lose blood, your body tries to shut off the blood supply to other parts of your body in order to maintain blood flow to your brain. When there is shortage of glucose, your body tries to restrict supply exclusively to the brain.

When any disease process changes your brain function, it is an indicator of the dire stress your body is undergoing. As you get older, it takes less and less to produce cloudy thinking and confusion because your body loses the ability to properly respond to physiological stress over time.

When you have an infection, you develop a fever, and your heart rate goes up. You get chills or rigors that are your body's way of showing inflammation and activating your immune system. In someone of advanced age, the body's response to infection is blunted. The adaptive mechanism and immune system is unable to mount the normal reaction of inflammation and fever. In elderly patients, cloudy thinking is often the first sign of physiological stress in the body.

Unfortunately, people often seem to think that it is normal for elderly people to get a little confused now and then and may not pay attention to a change in mental status. It is true that the prevalence of dementia is higher in older individuals, but any sudden change in mental status is not normal. That's why it's important to have the background information about a person's baseline mental status when evaluating any change. If you know that a loved one does not have a history of dementia and does not normally get confused, you need to clearly communicate that to the ER physician. You need to be as specific as possible to avoid any doubts. Tell the doctor how your loved one behaves normally, how he or she reads newspapers or does crossword puzzles, how active he or she is in the community, and what kind of indoor and outdoor activities he or she engages in. When you clearly communicate the baseline function level of an elderly family member, you provide the background information used to determine both the diagnosis and treatment.

Organ System: The Brain

Your brain is a very active organ that needs a significant amount of blood flow and nutrients. It is the control and command center of your body. You will learn more about specific parts of the brain and their significance in the next chapter.

7. The Speech Has It

How Stacy's Confused Speech Spoke Volumes about Her Condition

When someone is not talking straight, closer examination of the speech is necessary to untangle the problem.

When Stacy was admitted to the hospital with pneumonia, her case seemed simple. All she seemed to need was medication. The only reason she couldn't go home was that she was a little short of breath and required oxygen. Two or three days, and she would be out, her doctor said.

Little did Stacy know that the next three days in the hospital would be anything but simple.

The last few days had been a rollercoaster. On her first night in the hospital, a nurse had discovered that Stacy's blood sugar was extremely high. By the next morning, it had been determined that she had diabetes. While she was still reeling from the news, Stacy got some more bad news. Her blood pressure was running high. That night, she had to take intravenous blood-pressure medication. There was more bad news: Stacy's cholesterol was sky-high as well, and the doctor believed all her symptoms were related to her weight. He said she needed to lose at least thirty pounds.

Stacy was frustrated. She almost regretted coming to the hospital, much less staying the past few nights. She wanted the doctor to leave her alone, but she shied away from the confrontation. Instead she began to complain to the nurse about small things—the food, the bed, noise in the hallway, and bad smells. She was so upset that she couldn't sleep. That night, the nurse offered her a sleeping pill, which she refused. She'd heard about people getting hooked on sleeping pills. However, after lying in bed for hours, she accepted a sleeping pill after 3:00 a.m. By 4:00 a.m., she was asleep until 7:00 a.m., when the doctor started making his rounds. Upset and groggy, the last thing Stacy wanted to hear was a lecture from a doctor about her blood pressure, diabetes, cholesterol, and weight. She just wanted to be left alone to sleep, but that didn't seem possible. Nurses were constantly coming into Stacy's room. One would prick her finger to check her blood-sugar levels. Another would check her blood pressure every hour. They all reminded her to keep the oxygen tube in her nose, which was very uncomfortable, but it would keep her from developing a collapsed lung on top of her pneumonia. EKGs, x-rays, and all kinds of blood tests seemed to be constant. A dietician came to discuss her diet and her weight, which were affecting her lung expansion. A social worker came to discuss her insurance and what might and might not be covered. By her third night, Stacy didn't care about her recovery. She just wanted to get out of the hospital at any cost. When a nurse suggested that she get more exercise at the hospital by walking around, Stacy couldn't take it anymore.

"Seriously?" she demanded. "You want me to get up and walk? At this rate, I'll keep on walking right out the door. I just can't take this anymore. I'm sick and tired of hearing what's good for me. You don't know me. What I need is rest, at home and in my own bed. Please just give me my clothes. I need to get out of here."

"Stacy, I'm so sorry," the nurse said, shocked. "I know it can be stressful to be in a hospital. I'm sorry if I pushed you too much. I only said those things so that you could get better sooner and get home sooner. I'm sorry. You just take your time."

Stacy looked into the nurse's eyes, realizing that the nurse was only trying to help. She burst into tears.

"No, I'm sorry. I know you were only trying to help me. I'm just so frustrated. It's just one thing after another. I just turned fifty, my kids just started college, and my husband just lost his job. Now I'm finding out I have all sorts of health problems, and I just don't know how to handle any of this."

The nurse asked if Stacy would take antianxiety medication, and Stacy accepted gratefully. The nurse left to call the doctor to authorize antianxiety medication. When he heard that Stacy's vitals were relatively stable, except for her blood pressure, and that she was on two liters of oxygen, saturating at 95 percent, he agreed. He instructed the nurse to give Stacy one milligram of Ativan by mouth every four hours as needed.

The nurse gave Stacy the antianxiety medication, and it started working within twenty minutes. Stacy felt calm and sleepy. She dozed for the next three hours before the nurse interrupted her sleep to give her some IV medication. Stacy's blood pressure was just too high. The nurse had to give her some IV medications. This time, Stacy complied without complaint.

"Thank you, Stacy," the nurse said. "Can you tell me your full name and date of birth? I'm sorry, but I'm required to ask this before giving you this medication."

Stacy answered dutifully. After the nurse gave her the medication, Stacy began to feel strange. "I was feeling better after you gave me that...that...what do you call it? That...thing that I swallowed."

"The anxiety pill?" the nurse suggested.

"Yes, that. That thing made me sleepy and calm. But this thing in my...what do you call it? Well, my...my...well...my...this part." Stacy pointed at her arm.

"Your arm?" the nurse said.

"Yes, yes that thing on my...that part...started squeezing me. I feel a little tense in my...well...right...there." Stacy pointed to her forehead.

"Stacy, are you feeling all right?"

"Yes, I'm fine...I just have a little tightness in my...well...up there."

"Your forehead?" the nurse prompted.

"Yes, that's it, forehead. Did my...my...what do you call him...the man I'm married to...my, my...him, did he call?"

"Your husband? Yes, he called earlier. I didn't want to wake you up because you were finally sound asleep. But Stacy I'm worried about you. You seem confused."

"No, no I'm fine. That thing you gave me earlier helped. I feel better."

"Well, I will just call the doctor and make sure you're all right."

She left to call the doctor, who suggested the Ativan or lack of sleep might be making Stacy confused. Still, the nurse wasn't convinced. Stacy's language was muddled in an uncharacteristic way. When she explained that Stacy had referred to her husband as "that him," the doctor was concerned. He thanked the nurse and headed down to see Stacy. When he sat down with Stacy, he began to ask questions that led to a very distressing conversation.

"Hi Stacy, how are you feeling?"

"I'm fine. Thank you."

"I'm glad, Stacy. Can you tell me where you are?"

"Well, I'm here. What do you mean by that? I'm in the place where you go when you are sick."

"Yes, Stacy, but can you tell me what this placed is called?"

"Yes, yes, of course I know what they call this place...the...the...place for sick people. The...you know what I mean."

71

"Yes, I do, but would you tell me what you call this place?"

"Of course, yes, it's the...the...I'm sorry. I don't know what's wrong with me. I can't seem to remember the word."

The doctor was very concerned. He took a pen out of his pocked and held it out to Stacy. "Can you tell me what this is?" he asked.

"Of course. It's a...well...the thing you write with."

"And this?" The doctor pointed to the bed. "Can you tell me what this is?"

"It's the thing you sleep on. This one isn't very comfortable, but it's where I've been sleeping."

"Stacy, I'm very concerned about you." The doctor frowned. "I need to do a full neurological exam on you."

The doctor started by checking her eyes. He then asked her to smile and grin. He asked her to stick her tongue out and puff out her cheeks. He asked her to scrunch her eyebrows together. He asked her to grip his fingers. He asked her to raise her hands. He asked her to stand up and walk a few steps.

Stacy was able to do all those things without any problem. Next, the doctor conducted what he called a mini mental test—a series of questions. After the test, it was clear that Stacy had one specific problem: she couldn't name things, even familiar things. She could describe an object, but she couldn't remember its name. The doctor was worried. He suspected Stacy had experienced a mini stroke. Stacy needed a CT scan of her head right away, he said.

But the CT scan came back normal. When Stacy heard the news, she was confused.

"Is this good news?" she asked.

"Well, you show no signs of bleeding, but you probably had a small stroke."

"But—" Stacy hesitated, "I thought everything looked normal."

"The CT scan does look normal, but it would be normal if you had a small stroke like this. I ordered the CT scan because I wanted to make sure you had no bleeding in your head. I'm going to order a few tests in the morning to try to find out what caused your stroke. I'll also order an MRI of your brain to see if we can see the actual stroke. The MRI is more sensitive to a stroke, even when it is very small. In the meantime, I'll start you on medication to help prevent further strokes."

"Will I get back to normal?" Stacy was worried.

"There's a good chance that you may have a complete recovery, but it may take some time. It's hard to predict how long that may be. I'll have a speech therapist evaluate you in the morning as well. She'll be able to formulate a long-term rehab plan and exercises to help you recover your speech."

"Thanks," Stacy sighed. "Can you turn off that thing? It's too bright."

"Yes," the doctor said. "I'll turn off the light. You get some rest."

The next morning, Stacy was wheeled down to the radiology department for the MRI of her brain. The technicians checked Stacy to make sure she had no metal objects on her person, like jewelry.

An MRI operates with very strong magnetic fields. Any loose metal object within the perimeter of the field would be attracted to the magnetic field and could act as a dangerous projectile. An MRI (Magnetic Resonance Imaging) works by sending very strong magnetic fields and radio waves to our body. The hydrogen atoms in your body resonate in the presence of strong magnetism and send out radio signals. These radio signals are analyzed by the MRI machine. The computer then forms images from these signals, and they are displayed on the screen. An MRI can take more detailed images of soft tissues than a CT scan because it works with hydrogen atoms that are abundant in water. It does not require dense material to create the images like traditional x-ray machines do.

When the MRI results came back, they presented fewer answers than the doctor had hoped. Stacy had a small area on the left side of her brain that seemed to have an abnormal signal, suggesting a new stroke. The ultrasound of her heart was normal. An ultrasound of major arteries in her neck showed some plaque and some narrowing on Stacy's arteries, but it did not show any major blockage that could cause such a stroke. After all the tests were done, the doctor was not able to find any specific reason for the stroke. He concluded that the stroke was caused by the combination of diabetes, high blood pressure, and high cholesterol. He emphasized to Stacy that she needed to keep her blood pressure under control. She would need to take her medications regularly. When she was discharged, Stacy still had significant trouble finding words, but she did learn to adapt.

Teaching Points

Basic Approach: Speech Problems

When someone isn't speaking rationally or appears confused or different, it is important to seek medical attention right away. The difference between types of confusion and speech abnormalities can be very subtle, but it's important to distinguish between them as each can have consequences.

When your speech is confused, all aspects of thinking and memory are impaired. You may not know where you are, what you are doing, or what is happening around you. You may have a selective loss of memory, remembering things from the distant past but not recent memory. This kind of general confusion is mainly associated with diseases that affect the whole body and also cause problems with proper brain function.

When you have a specific type of speech problem like Stacy's, the problem is more likely to be a stroke or disease related to a specific part of the brain. Other specific speech problems include loss of fluency, difficulty understanding language, trouble repeating instructions, slowing of speech, and difficulty forming a structured sentence. On the surface, people with all these conditions appear confused and nonsensical. If you notice a speech problem in a loved one, know that you do not need to figure out what specific type of speech problem he or she has. If you can distinguish between the general confusion and specific speech problem, you can already make a huge difference. A common example of generalized confusion is urine infection in the elderly, as described in chapter 6. A specific speech problem most commonly suggests stroke.

Organ system: The Brain and the Nervous System

Your brain is a very complex organ. As a command and control center of the whole body, your brain has different areas that control different parts of your body and coordinate a myriad of bodily functions. It has millions of connective nerves that link one part of the brain to another, consuming a significant amount of energy.

Because of this highly complex organization of the brain, symptoms arising from dysfunction of the brain can present in complex and bizarre ways. To understand the different types of symptoms from brain dysfunction, you can look at several different categories of brain function. The first is the higher cognitive function, which people normally associate with the brain. It includes thinking, memory, learning, and language. The second type of brain function is movement and coordination. The third type is less obvious: your brain controls almost every internal organ in your body on some level. This control is asserted without any conscious action or knowledge on your part by the autonomic unconscious brain. Your brain is also the processing center of all your senses, and it is what allows you to see, hear, feel, or smell something. Your brain also processes emotions and makes you feel happy, sad, angry, or excited.

Modern neuroscience has identified and studied different parts of the brain that are associated with different functions. They have mapped the regions of the brain that control different parts of the body when you move. They have identified areas of the brain that make you remember things. They have also mapped the areas of the brain that makes you feel the emotions that you experience in life. However, as your knowledge of different parts of the brain grows, you also realize that all these parts are connected and that they work together in a very complicated way. There is still so much to learn, and every new discovery leads to many new horizons to explore.

For practical purposes, you need to able to distinguish between two different types of brain function: global and focal. A focal brain symptom denotes an actual disease inside a known part of the brain. The most common disease causing focal brain dysfunction is a stroke.

Global brain dysfunction causes generalized symptoms. In other words, these are symptoms you cannot pinpoint to a particular location and region of the brain. Most global brain dysfunction is caused by an incident occurring outside of the brain, influencing the whole brain. Significant chemical imbalance, high levels of toxins, overwhelming infection, an abnormally active immune system, and very high blood pressure are a few examples of factors that can have a generalized impact on the whole brain. People with generalized brain dysfunction may have generalized weakness, trouble walking, generalized confusion, disorientation, trouble with memory and concentration, and other similar symptoms. A person who is intoxicated with high blood-alcohol levels is a perfect example of someone experiencing global brain dysfunction. In this case, the cause of dysfunction is high level of a particular toxin (alcohol).

On the other hand, focal (isolated) brain dysfunction causes very complex and bizarre symptoms. It may only affect movement, sensation, or balance, either in the whole body or in a particular region. The symptoms appear to be very strange and illogical to you, but they follow a predictable sequence in the brain for a neurologist. Based on symptoms, a neurologist can predict which region of the brain may have been affected. It is not possible for you to learn to relate your symptoms to a part of your brain, but you can learn to distinguish between global and focal symptoms.

Someone who is drunk is an example of global brain dysfunction. But if someone starts to walk as though intoxicated without any other drunken behavior, focal dysfunction is occurring in the part of the brain that controls balance and coordination.

Someone lying on the bed, confused and weak, has global brain dysfunction. But someone with weakness in the right leg, right arm, and left side of the face has a focal brain dysfunction. In this case, the pattern of weakness follows a known brain anatomy.

Someone who is heavily sedated in the hospital has global brain dysfunction because he or she is unable to open his or her eyes or to see or to feel. Someone who has healthy, normal eyes but is unable to see has a focal dysfunction based in the part of the brain that helps you process the signals coming from the eyes.

As I stated earlier, the most common disease causing focal brain dysfunction is a stroke. The brain needs a rich supply of blood to function properly, and there is an extensive network of arteries that supply blood to the different parts of the brain. These arteries originate in the heart and climb up the neck to go inside the brain. Once inside, they branch out, supplying blood to all the nooks and grooves of the brain. Many important areas get blood from more than one branch to protect them in case one of the branches gets clogged. The pattern of blood flow to the brain and areas supplied by major branches is well known in neuroscience.

A stroke occurs when the blood supply to part of the brain gets interrupted. Symptoms of a stroke are always focal because they affect certain parts of the brain. When you understand what focal brain dysfunction looks like, you can quickly recognize stroke-like symptoms and seek timely help.

8. Something Popped

*How Seth's Description of His Pain Helped His Doctor
Solve a Mystery*

*Better diagnosis of chest pain lies in the specifics of the
symptoms. Analysis of how a patient feels will help form
a better diagnosis than will a categorization of
symptoms.*

This morning, like every other morning for the past two
months, college junior Seth got up at six o'clock to go
for a run. He had been training for the marathon with
friends, and the big run was just one week away now.
He'd had a cold for the past week and was only just
getting back up to speed, but he was excited nonetheless.
Since Seth had been healthy all his life, with no major
illnesses or hospitalizations except for appendicitis at the
age of fourteen, no one would have expected where
Seth's run abruptly ended that day.

After running for thirty minutes, Seth stopped to
drink some water and then resumed his pace. Five
minutes in, he felt as though something in his body
popped. He stopped in the middle of the track and lay
down. The pain was unbearable, especially on the right
side of his chest. He felt like he was running out of
breath. He tried to get up but found he could only sit up
very slowly. Reaching into his pocket with great
difficulty, Seth dialed 911 and called for help.

When the paramedics arrived, Seth's vitals checked
out fine, except for a high respiratory rate. Even with a
finger sensor, his oxygen saturation was fine. The
paramedics gave him oxygen but only because his
distressed state seemed to be interfering with his
breathing. He was still complaining of severe pain on the
right side of his chest, though, so the paramedics laid

him on a stretcher and wheeled him out to the ambulance, where they attached leads to his chest for an EKG. The machine read the EKG as normal, but the information was still faxed to the nearest emergency department to be reviewed by the ER doctor, along with the message that they had a twenty-two-year-old male with chest pain arriving in five minutes.

Five minutes later, Seth was transferred from the ambulance to a gurney and then to a hospital bed. He was in a lot of pain, but his vital signs were still normal. The oxygen tube was still in his nose, and his oxygen saturation was registered at 98 percent. He appeared to be breathing fast and shallow.

"Did you have any similar chest pain in the past?" the ER doctor asked Seth.

"No," Seth said, "nothing like this ever happened to me in the past."

"Any heart disease or heart problems that you know of?"

"No, nothing that I have been told of."

"Any lung problems?"

"No, I have been very healthy as far as I can tell. I don't remember being in the hospital since my appendix surgery when I was fourteen."

"Do you smoke cigarettes?" the doctor glanced up from Seth's chart.

Seth shook his head. "Never."

"Does your family have a history of heart or lung problems?"

"My grandpa died of a heart attack when he was seventy-eight."

The doctor listened to Seth's chest with a stethoscope. "Take a few deep breaths," he instructed. Seth breathed in and out and then stopped abruptly.

"Wow, that hurts," Seth said, wincing. "The right upper side of my chest hurts, like some sharp knife cutting my chest every time I take a deep breath like that."

The doctor finished his physical exam as quickly as possible to avoid any further pain. He then scribbled some orders on Seth's chart and spoke to the nurse. "Seth is in a lot of pain," he explained. "I ordered a morphine shot for him, so please give it to him as soon as possible. Also, take him to radiology for a chest x-ray as soon as you are done with the morphine. I've also ordered some blood tests, but they can wait until the x-ray is done."

The nurse injected four milligrams of morphine into Seth's IV line. Within five minutes, it started working. Seth was still feeling the pain, but it was much more bearable. A nurse helped Seth into a wheelchair and took him downstairs to get an x-ray.

In the radiology department, the radiology technician greeted Seth and asked him for his name and date of birth. Seth told him, and the technician nodded. "Well," he said, "the doctor seems to have ordered a full upright x-ray. You need to be able to stand still for a few minutes for this x-ray. Do you think you can do that?"

"I think so. Yes." Seth stood up and leaned his chest against the plate of the machine just like the technician told him to. He had to take a deep breath and hold it for a few seconds. It was painful, but he was able to finish the test without any problems.

When Seth returned to the ER, a lab technician was waiting there to draw some blood. As soon as the lab technician went out, the doctor came back in. Seth was surprised to see the doctor back so soon—did that mean bad news?

"Well, I just looked at the chest x-ray," the doctor paused.

"And?" Seth needed to know.

"Well, I saw some air that was leaking out of your right lung."

"What?" Seth asked. "How can air be leaking out of one of my lungs? Don't people breathe air in and out of their lungs?"

"Don't worry. I'll explain it to you. Bear with me for a while." The doctor went to the whiteboard in the room and drew a picture of the chest cavity with two lungs in it. "This is how normal lungs appear," he said, pointing. "Each lung is lined by a thin layer of membrane like a plastic sheet. The same plastic-like sheet folds back on itself and lines the inner walls of your chest. There is a small amount of lubricant in between these two membranes. Your lungs expand and collapse when you breathe in and out. This lubricant prevents injury to your lungs from this constant movement. Now here is what happened to the right side of your lung." He wiped off the upper third of the right lung and redrew the membranes over the remaining part. "Somehow some air leaked out of this side of your lung, and now that air is trapped between these two membranes. The pocket of air has pushed down on your right lung, and now your lung can only expand about to two-thirds of its capacity. When you take a deep breath, your lungs try to expand more to create some pressure on the membrane next to the air pocket. This is why it hurts so much when you take deep breaths."

"Wow." Seth looked down at his hands, shaking his head. After a moment, he looked up. "So," he ventured hesitantly, "what happens now?"

"Well," the doctor said matter-of-factly, "let's look at this drawing again. We need to extract the air from this air pocket to allow your lungs to expand fully. The best way to do this is to insert a small tube into the air pocket that can slowly suck the air out. Since the tube will need to be an effective one-way valve, we'll connect the tube with a suction pump that will provide a low, constant, and controlled suction force."

"That sounds kind of scary. Will it hurt?"

"It hurts a little bit as we put the tube in, but we'll numb the area before we insert it. You may still feel some pain, but we will give you IV shots for the pain as you need them. If you're ready, I'll call the cardio-thoracic surgeon. He's very experienced. He should be here within the next thirty minutes, and we'll keep the oxygen on until he arrives. Don't hesitate to tell the nurse if your pain gets worse again."

Knowing there was a cure for his condition made Seth feel a bit better, but he still didn't understand why the air bubble had formed in the first place. He suddenly realized he had a billion different questions. "How did this happen? I mean, why did my lung start leaking air, just like that? Will it happen again? Will I ever be able to run a marathon again?"

"Well," the doctor said, nodding, "there are some lung diseases that can cause air leakage, but in your case, I don't see any signs of other lung disease. I think you probably have what we call a primary spontaneous pneumothorax. It's rare—it happens to approximately ten to twenty males out of one hundred thousand. It seems like young, tall male athletes like you happen to get this more frequently than others. There are many theories about why it happens to this demographic, but none of them have been confirmed. The surgeon may have more specific information about when you can start running again, but I think it's safe to say that you'll need to take it easy for a few weeks. I can't promise, of course, but I think you will eventually recover from this and be able to run the marathon again. Again, I can't make any promises, but I would look forward to seeing you run the marathon next year. Now, there is a chance that this might happen again. If it happens more than once, your cardio-thoracic surgeon may perform a surgical procedure to prevent a relapse. Since this is your first time, however, I believe just a chest tube and a day or two in the hospital for observation will probably be all you need."

Seth was admitted to the hospital after successful placement of the chest tube in the emergency department. A small tube coming out of his right side drained small amounts of air a little bit at a time. With his pain kept under control with a morphine IV, Seth fell asleep early that night and slept deeply.

The next morning, Seth woke up breathing easier. He still felt some pain, but it was tolerable. The surgeon who had operated on him was just making his rounds. Approaching Seth, he smiled. "How are you feeling now, Seth?" the surgeon asked.

"Good. My chest still hurts a little, but not as much as yesterday."

"Great," the surgeon said, nodding. "Let me listen to your lungs now." He put his stethoscope on the back of Seth's chest and told him to take a few deep breaths. He listened patiently for a few minutes and compared the sounds coming out of Seth's lungs on the right side with the sounds coming from the left. He also tapped both lungs with his fingers and noted the difference in percussive tones.

Seth's collapsed lung had healed significantly by the third day of his hospital stay. There was just a small trace of air on the topmost part of the lung. Eventually the surgeon removed the tube and observed Seth for two hours after. When Seth's stable condition was confirmed, he was discharged. He thanked his ER doctor, adding that he hoped to see him at the marathon next year.

Teaching Points

Basic Approach: Chest Pain

At the end of chapter 3, you learned about chest pain in the context of a heart attack. However, not all chest pain is caused by heart attacks. In this chapter and in chapter 11, you will learn about other causes of chest pain and learn several key things to remember about it.

As you know by now, the greater amount of detail you provide on any symptom, the easier it becomes to identify the correct diagnosis. This is never truer than when it comes to chest pain.

In chapter 3, you learned how your heart does not have nerve fibers that can directly transport pain sensations to your brain. Now you'll learn about organs and structures inside your chest that have pain nerves that connect directly to your brain.

Your chest wall, ribs, the lining of your lungs and of the heart, and major blood vessels are the important places inside your chest that have plenty of pain-sensing nerves that conduct signals directly to your brain. These nerves are very similar to those located in your skin. The pain originating in these places can be fairly sharp and localized, unlike the dull, achy, vaguely localized pain that comes from a heart attack.

Pain originating in your lungs has to cause irritation or pressure on the lining of your lungs for you to feel it. Any inflammation in your lungs that spreads out and reaches the lung lining will cause pain. This type of pain usually worsens when you cough or take a deep breath because the lining of your lungs stretches when you do so. When air leaks out into the space between the two linings of the lungs, it puts pressure on the linings.

Besides leaked air, there are a number of other diseases that can cause a similar type of pain in the chest. When you have an infection in your lungs (pneumonia), the inflammation can spread out to the lining of your lungs and can cause similar chest pain.

85

However, the inflammation spreads out slowly in pneumonia, and the onset of pain is gradual. You can also have similar pain from lung cancer. However, you may have lung cancer growing inside your lungs for a long time without causing any pain. If the cancer grows without touching the lining of your lungs, it can be painless. Once it grows out and touches the lining, it causes unrelenting, sharp pain in your chest. Similar pain can be caused by a blood clot in the lungs if the affected area involves or is in close proximity to the lining of the lungs. The symptoms of blood clots in your lungs can also have rapid onset, just like the symptoms of leaked air, but the pain is not as severe or dramatic.

Sharp pain in the chest that worsens with coughing or deep breathing indicates irritation of the lining of the lungs. With this kind of pain, the likelihood of a heart attack is low, but you may have an equally life-threatening problem that needs immediate medical attention. Remember that the exact description of how your pain started is very important in diagnosing the cause of the pain. In this case, what Seth felt was exactly what happened to his lung: he felt something pop, and as his lung leaked air, he felt as though he was running out of gas.

9. Seeing Red

How Throwing Up Blood Was a Wake-Up Call for Yolanda

The reason a patient throws up blood can be found in the details of what happened before the blood appeared.

It was six in the morning when paramedics wheeled Yolanda into the ER. She was sobbing, tears running down her face to mix with blood on her lips. Yolanda had been celebrating her twenty-first birthday the night before. She was the last of her friends to turn twenty-one, and her friends had been planning her birthday party for a while. In the past, she'd had one or two drinks at a party—an occasional margarita or a beer or two—but she had never had more than that.

The night of her birthday, Yolanda's best friend threw a huge party in the basement of her townhouse, where they could play the music loudly. It was a fun party, and Yolanda's friends made her feel like it was all about her. She was finally old enough to drink as much as she wanted. She didn't have to rely on her friends to sneak her alcohol anymore. Everyone was having a good time, and someone suggested tequila shots. At first, the liquor was too harsh for Yolanda, and she didn't want to drink anymore. Her friends wouldn't take no for an answer, though, and insisted that she do a shot every time her best friend did one. She finally gave in and started matching her friends, shot for shot. Soon she lost count of how many she had.

Yolanda woke up around five o'clock the next morning, confused. She was in her apartment, although she couldn't remember how she got there. She was still very drunk, and the night was a blur. She was still wearing last night's clothes. She tried to get up, but she was too weak and dizzy. She slowly dragged herself into the bathroom and was disgusted by what she saw. There was vomit everywhere, and the stench was unbearable.

She started getting sick again. As she vomited, her stomach ached, and her esophagus burned. She tried to stop but found she couldn't control her retching. She kept vomiting, even though there was nothing in her stomach to bring up. With every dry heave, her stomach and esophagus contracted violently, every attempt stronger than the one before. Frightened, she realized that she was starting to make loud noises as she retched. Her stomach felt extremely sore, and all of a sudden, there was bright-red blood flushing out of her mouth.

Yolanda was terrified. Was she going to die? All she had wanted to do was have some fun on her birthday. She looked at the floor and saw her cell phone by the sink. She grabbed it and called 911.

At the ER, a nurse settled Yolanda in a room and checked her vitals, which all appeared to be normal with the exception of her 120 heart rate. Her heart was beating too fast. The nurse told her that she needed to calm down and wait for the doctor. When the doctor arrived, Yolanda told him that she was dying and that she was going to bleed to death.

"Yolanda, you're not dying," the doctor said. "Your vitals are stable, but I do need you to relax and tell me exactly what happened."

Yolanda nodded and said she'd do her best, but she was fighting back tears. When she was finally able to tell the doctor what had happened, he had questions about the night.

"So how much blood do you think you may have thrown up so far?" the doctor asked, concerned.

"I don't know. Too much."

"Would you say more than ten cups?" he asked, holding up the plastic cup next to Yolanda's hospital bed.

"No," Yolanda shook her head. "Not that much."

"More than…five cups?"

"Probably not, but more than two."

"OK, so you lost anywhere between two and five cups of blood. Does that sound about right?"

"I guess so," Yolanda mumbled, embarrassed.

The doctor then examined her quickly and scribbled on the chart. "All right, no need to worry. The nurses here will take good care of you. I've ordered some medications, some blood tests, and x-rays. But the nurse needs to get an IV line in your arm so that we can give you an antinausea medication. You just relax here, and I will back once I have some test results."

When the doctor left, Yolanda started crying again. After a few tries, the nurse was able to finally get some blood flowing out from her veins and into the needle. Yolanda's dehydration made her blood flow sluggish and difficult to tap. The nurse then inserted the small plastic tube into the vein to maintain intravenous access. As soon as the IV was ready, she injected an antinausea medication into Yolanda's veins. A few minutes later, she gave her a shot of morphine, followed by eighty milligrams of IV pantoprazole, a medicine to decrease the amount of acid in the stomach and reduce the risk of bleeding in the stomach. Reducing the acid level would also help with the burning pain Yolanda had from prolonged vomiting and dry heaving.

Within thirty minutes, the doctor came back with test results in his hand. Yolanda wasn't doing as bad as she felt. Her blood count was still within normal range. Her body was definitely dehydrated, but her kidney function was normal. Her blood-alcohol level was still high, but her liver enzymes were normal.

"Doctor, if everything looks great…why do I feel like I'm dying?" she asked.

"Well, you had a binge-drinking episode. You probably drank too much, too fast. You are not a habitual drinker. Your body could not adjust to the very high level of alcohol in your blood, and you got very sick. You woke up with severe nausea and vomiting. Your nausea worsened when you smelled the vomit from last night, and that made you even sicker. You dry heaved so hard that you probably tore up your esophagus."

"How do you know all this? From the blood tests?" Yolanda looked relieved.

"Well, not just from the blood tests. We still need to confirm with further testing, but I've given you my working diagnosis. You forcefully vomited about two cups of blood after a night of drinking. Your blood work did not show any signs of liver damage or kidney damage. The most likely cause of bleeding in this situation is tearing of the esophagus. Now do you have any other questions for me? If not, the nurse will arrange a bed for you upstairs."

"No questions." Yolanda shook her head. "Thank you for helping me. I was so scared."

In the next thirty minutes, Yolanda was taken upstairs to the third floor of the hospital. Her nurse came and sat with her. She had tons of questions for Yolanda and logged Yolanda's answers on a computer. When she was finished, she left to get a doctor.

A new doctor came in and asked Yolanda all the same questions the ER doctor had asked. It was frustrating to repeat everything, but Yolanda was too polite to say as much. She didn't want to put her doctor off, so she went through the whole ordeal one more time and went through what happened.

"Thank you for giving me all the details. I'm going to continue the IV medicine to keep your stomach-acid level down. I also want to give your stomach and your food pipe some rest, though, so I'm afraid you will have to hold off on any food or water until you get better. You may have a small tear in your esophagus as per your previous doctor's diagnosis, but there are some other possibilities that I want to be sure to rule out." The doctor explained that Yolanda could have some underlying problems that might have worsened with the drinking, like an ulcer or another preexisting stomach problem. It could have been made worse by excessive drinking or the stress of a hangover and vomiting.

"So how do we make sure?" Yolanda asked. She was exhausted.

"We need to take a look. I will let you rest for a day with medications and IV fluids. Then I'll call in one of our specialists to perform a procedure to look inside your esophagus, stomach, and the upper part of your intestine. The procedure is called an upper endoscopy. It involves numbing your throat, inserting a tube with a camera into your mouth, and gently pushing it toward your stomach. The specialist will be watching everything directly on a video monitor as she guides the camera in and closely inspects the lining of your food pipe, stomach, and intestine. She can also see if anything is still bleeding. The tip of the tube will also have tools to take a small sample of your tissue. She can do a biopsy and examine the lining of your stomach under a microscope and find out if there is anything else going on at the tissue and cellular level."

"Will it hurt?"

"It will be uncomfortable, but not too painful. You'll be sedated the entire time. I know it sounds daunting, but we need to find out the exact cause of your bleeding, and this is the way to do it. You don't have to undergo the procedure, but I do strongly recommend it. I will give you some written information about the procedure, and you can do your own research. When you're ready, just let me know if you want the procedure. We won't do anything unless you are comfortable with it."

"I'm just a little scared," Yolanda admitted. "Could anything go wrong with the procedure?"

The doctor explained that any medical procedure had some risks, but that an upper endoscopy was a fairly routine procedure. There was still a small chance of complications—more bleeding, more tearing, or a possible infection—but the chances were very low. The scopes were very sophisticated, and the surgeon was very skilled. Yolanda still seemed hesitant, so the doctor repeated his earlier offer. "I can't stress this enough, though. If you're hesitant, please read up on the procedure, and do your own research before you decide. I'll give you a printout on endoscopy and its complications. You can also find more information on the Internet. If you have any further questions, I'll be happy to answer those for you."

Yolanda thanked the doctor. When he left, she called her friend and asked her to bring her laptop to the hospital. She was feeling much better by now, although she was still nauseous. *As long as I'm not dry heaving anymore,* she thought.

She read the patient education material given to her by the doctor and started researching the procedure on her laptop. She did a web search for the term "Mallory-Weiss Tear" and found several websites describing the disease. She read several articles and realized that the diagnosis made sense.

She was not sure if she really needed the endoscopy or not. Most of the articles she read said that endoscopy could be done to confirm the diagnosis but did not say if she really needed it. She was scared of the thought of having a tube, much less a camera, inside her stomach.

She did a search for "potential problems from endoscopy" and read several articles about the risks and complications. She also found an online forum where patients described their experiences with the procedure. After weighing all the information she had collected, Yolanda decided to go through with the procedure. The doctor was pleased and scheduled the endoscopy for the following afternoon.

The next day, the results of the endoscopy were good. The procedure had revealed that there was indeed a small tear in Yolanda's esophagus, and it was already healing. The specialist saw no other abnormality and was confident that the tear would continue to heal without any complications. The admitting doctor told Yolanda that she could start drinking some clear liquids that night if she felt like it. The nurse brought her a piece of Jell-O, and she ate it without any problems, although her appetite wasn't particularly strong, and she was very, very tired.

The day after that, Yolanda woke up feeling much better after a restorative night's sleep. She was refreshed and starving. After some chicken soup, she felt even better. After hearing from her doctor that she could go home, Yolanda felt her best yet.

The doctor felt confident releasing her, but he still had a warning or two. Yolanda would need to rest up for a couple of days and slowly advance her diet. If she didn't have any pain, nausea, or vomiting, she could gradually work up to eating normally again. But under no circumstances should she drink too much alcohol. Yolanda assured him that drinking was the last thing on her mind.

Teaching Points

Basic Approach: Vomiting Blood

Vomiting blood is always a medical emergency. It does not matter how it happened or what caused it—you need to go the emergency department right away. The cause and seriousness of the condition cannot be determined just by the amount of blood or the details of your story. Medical professionals need to watch you closely to make sure it is not a life-threatening medical emergency.

Having said that, your story of how you ended up throwing up blood helps the doctor make some educated guess about the cause of your bleeding. It helps him or her formulate the best treatment plan.

Organ System: The Liver and Upper GI Tract

The gastrointestinal (GI) tract starts at the mouth and ends at the anus. The upper part of the GI tract runs from the mouth, to the throat, to the esophagus (food pipe), to the stomach, and to the upper part of the small intestine. Vomiting blood can be a sign of bleeding in any of these places.

The esophagus has a rich supply of blood vessels and is a common site of bleeding. Somewhat elastic, the esophagus can expand to accommodate food when you swallow. It also has muscles that produce a contraction rhythm that pushes food down into your stomach. It is easily enflamed by the reflux of food and acid in the stomach. Over time, this inflammation can erode the surface and expose blood vessels that can bleed. Mechanical stress, such as occurs when you force the esophagus to its limit by coughing too hard, retching too hard, or vomiting too many times, can also lead to bleeding. This is what happened to Yolanda.

The stomach is where food mixes with acid, which is very corrosive and can easily erode the stomach's wall. Your stomach has several adaptive mechanisms to protect itself from this erosion while utilizing acid to help digest the food you eat. The lining of the stomach produces a layer of mucous that covers the stomach's surface like the coating on a nonstick pan. It prevents the acid from penetrating the surface. The cells in the surface of the stomach are also packed tightly to prevent acid from getting inside just in case it comes down the layer of mucous. The stomach also makes new cells to replace and replenish the whole stomach's surface once every few days.

Despite all these protective measures, acid does go down to the surface and erode the stomach lining. Sometimes it penetrates deep enough to erode a blood vessel and causes bleeding. At other times, it can erode deeper and wider, causing an ulcer or a complete breakdown of the top protective layer. An ulcer exposes the deep layer of stomach, leaving it open to attack from the acid.

There are multiple causes of increased stomach acid and reduced protective measures. Certain pain medications, too much stress, too much alcohol, and smoking are the major culprits. The upper part of the intestine can also have the same kind of inflammation and erosion that happens in the stomach. The resulting blood can flow back to the stomach and come out as vomiting blood. Risk factors for this type of bleeding are similar to those for stomach bleeding.

If we look at all the things that can cause upper GI bleeding, it seems like alcohol is a factor in almost all types of bleeding we have discussed so far. That is why it is difficult to estimate the cause of bleeding when someone with heavy alcohol abuse starts throwing up blood. In many cases, doctors assume the worst-case scenario and make treatment plans based on that. Of course cancer can also be behind the erosion of blood vessels and GI bleeding.

Yolanda was not a habitual alcohol abuser. She just had a binge-drinking experience. From the story, it seemed like multiple vomiting and retching episodes during her bad hangover were the cause of her bleeding. She tore her food pipe by pushing it to the limit with her retching and vomiting—a bad hangover gone worse. While Yolanda was lucky, esophageal bleeding can have much more serious consequences. Variceal bleeding, which occurs in people with severe liver problems and often stems from alcohol abuse, has a significantly worse prognosis than any other type of bleeding in the GI tract.

ESOPHAGEL VARICES

MAINLY DUE TO LIVER CIRRHOSIS

10. Coming Up Red

*How Throwing Up Blood Was the Beginning of the End
for Simon*

*Learn the consequences of continuing to drink in spite of
liver failure, and find out the dangers of throwing up
blood in that context.*

Simon had been admitted to the hospital several times in
the last few weeks. Most of the ICU nurses were very
familiar with him. He had a serious alcohol problem—he
had been drinking almost two liters of vodka daily for
the last twenty years. His social and family life had been
virtually destroyed by his drinking. He'd been divorced
now for more than five years, and his wife had sole
custody of the children. He had visitation rights but
rarely saw his children; even kids don't want to see their
dad when he's drunk. Unable to hold down a steady job,
Simon worked odd jobs to fund his drinking and lived in
low-income housing, which he struggled to afford.
Multiple DUIs had cost him his driver's license.

On that particular day, he was very tired. He was
approaching his forty-second birthday. He had been
hired by a local contractor to work on a roofing project
for a new strip mall. It was a very demanding job for
Simon, but he needed money to pay his rent and to buy
vodka. He'd tried to stop drinking many times in the
past, but the last time he'd tried, he had almost died and
had ended up in the hospital. The doctors had been
forced to use heavy sedatives to keep him calm and
avoid seizures—sedatives so heavy that Simon could not
breathe on his own and had to be intubated and hooked
up to a ventilator. He stayed in the hospital for more than
two weeks.

When he initially realized he had a problem, Simon

tried several rehab programs, but he could never maintain sobriety for more than a few days. Five years ago, several doctors had told Simon that his drinking had damaged his liver. They'd warned him that his liver would fail if he continued to drink, but he was scared to quit because every time he tried, he got sick. He'd learned the hard way about withdrawal symptoms and didn't want to risk having seizures again. He still felt fine when he drank—but not for long. Soon he started to feel weak and tired throughout the day. His skin itched constantly, and it turned pale with a yellowish hue. Several tortuous-looking veins popped up on his chest and his stomach, which had become distended.

Still Simon did not seek help or try to quit. Instead he tried his best to mask his symptoms, trying to act normally during the day and drinking his vodka at night. He stopped going to bars and restaurants and started drinking exclusively alone at home. He had a friend who would give him a ride to and from work. On his way home, Simon would stop at the gas station near his apartment and buy vodka. As soon as he got home, he started drinking and drank until he finished his daily quota.

One day Simon woke up after a night of drinking feeling very, very sick. As he got up to go to the bathroom, he was dizzy. Lurching to the toilet, he tried to vomit, but there was no need to try. Almost effortlessly, bright-red blood came rushing out of his mouth, filling the whole toilet bowl. He felt as if he were going to die then and there. He curled up on the bathroom floor for a while, a trickle of blood still trailing from his mouth. When he felt he could move, he slowly crawled out of his bathroom and made it to his cell phone, which was lying on the floor next to his bed. He called 911, just barely able to explain that he was vomiting blood and needed help.

By the time paramedics arrived at his apartment, Simon was barely conscious. He was still breathing, but he did not have any energy left to talk or move. They checked his pulse. It was very faint. They checked his blood pressure. It was quite low, at 85/42. They quickly inserted an IV line in his arm for a saline infusion and put him on a stretcher to wheel him out to the ambulance. They called ahead to the ER, telling the doctor that they had a patient with active bleeding and low blood pressure. By this point, they couldn't communicate with Simon. He only mumbled incoherently.

As soon as they arrived at the ER, the paramedics took Simon to the resuscitation room, where a team started working on him. His blood pressure was still low, and he had some leftover blood in his mouth. A nurse put the saline bag under pressure and pumped as much fluid into Simon as quickly as they could. Meanwhile another nurse started a second IV line in Simon's other arm and drew blood for testing and for matching— Simon was probably going to need a blood transfusion.

As Simon became even more unresponsive and lethargic, they decided to intubate him to protect his airway. They pumped more fluids into his body to raise his blood pressure, infusing about three liters of saline within thirty minutes. Soon his blood pressure showed slight signs of improvement. In the meantime, results of his blood tests started to come back. They didn't look good.

Simon was experiencing severe liver failure. He couldn't stop bleeding because his blood was low on clotting factors. The liver makes the majority of clotting factors that circulate in the blood, which help clot blood when needed. Blood clots prevent excessive bleeding by reducing the flow of blood from the site where it is bleeding. When the liver is damaged, it cannot efficiently produce those clotting factors.

Simon's blood count was also very low. He had already lost a significant amount of blood, and he was still bleeding internally. The nurses had to transfuse blood immediately to stabilize Simon, otherwise he would bleed to death. Once the transfusion was performed, his blood pressure improved enough for transfer to the ICU.

In the ICU, Simon still required further blood transfusions. Still hooked up to a ventilator, Simon was given sedatives to prevent withdrawal seizures. His blood count only rose slightly after an infusion of four units of blood—he was still bleeding internally. The only way to stop the bleeding would be to locate the source of the blood. The nurses called the gastroenterologist, who prepared to do an endoscopy right there in the ICU room. She inserted the tube with the camera into Simon's mouth and slowly guided it down through his esophagus until she saw the source of the bleeding—the esophageal wall was oozing blood from a large, distended vein, which seemed to have burst.

The gastroenterologist was prepared for this. She had used a special endoscope with a tip that could remotely clamp, cut, and tie a band around the bleeding site. Looking at the camera footage on a monitor, she was finally able to clamp the vessel after several attempts and band it to stop further bleeding. The nurses continued with the blood transfusion, infusing a total of eight units of blood before Simon's blood count stabilized. They also transfused several units of fresh frozen plasma (FFP) to try to boost clotting factors in the blood.

Fresh frozen plasma is the watery liquid component in blood. It contains all the soluble proteins, enzymes, and other active chemicals. FFP is collected from blood donors and frozen immediately to preserve the active

100

proteins and enzymes. Among the active components of plasma, clotting factors are some of the most important elements. These clotting factors can temporarily help restore the clotting ability of blood.

Simon's blood count and blood pressure eventually stabilized, but not enough to take him off the ventilator. Nurses tried to decrease sedation so that Simon would be able to breathe on his own. However, as they decreased sedation, he showed signs of severe alcohol withdrawal, and they had to increase the sedation again to prevent seizures and other complications.

Simon remained on the ventilator for more than three weeks. He developed an infection in his lungs, requiring multiple IV antibiotics for treatment. A feeding tube had to be inserted through a hole in his stomach to provide nutrition. With the exception of a few hours every day, Simon was kept under steady sedation and always failed the ventilation test—he couldn't breathe on his own. After three weeks of antibiotics and nutrition, he was just barely able to breathe on his own but was too weak to even stand. He couldn't swallow food and still had to rely on the tube in his stomach for nutrition. Eventually he was transferred to a nursing home for rehab and physical therapy.

Teaching Points

Basic Approach: Bleeding from Liver Failure

As discussed in the previous chapter, heavy alcohol abuse can lead to internal bleeding. Simon, whose drinking led to liver damage, is an example of the catastrophic effects of prolonged alcohol abuse. Longtime alcoholics often exhibit further signs of liver failure, and the damage is advanced and irreversible. When they start to exhibit signs of liver failure, it's hard to treat and save them. The most important way to prevent death and disability in people with severe alcohol abuse is to identify them before they reach this state and save them from complete liver failure.

Organ System: The Liver

The liver is one of the most important organs in your body. In order to recognize symptoms of liver failure, you need to understand what your liver actually does. The liver is the biggest chemical factory in your body. It performs thousands of chemical reactions every day, creating and breaking down complex compounds based on the needs of the body. It can change fat to sugar, sugar to fat, protein to sugar, and use protein and sugar to make thousands of other chemicals.

The liver makes the majority of clotting factors, which are the compounds that circulate in the blood to help it clot when needed. When the liver starts to fail, production of clotting factors is one of the first processes to break down. Alcohol abusers with advanced liver failure, like Simon, have very low levels of clotting factors and are therefore very vulnerable to massive, life-threatening bleeding.

Your liver makes the majority of protein-based compounds that circulate in your blood. One such protein is albumin. Similar to the material found in egg whites, albumin has a very important function circulating in the body. It prevents water from leaking out of the blood vessels. When you have a normal, healthy level of albumin inside your blood vessels, it attracts water molecules so that they can't escape. When the level of albumin decreases, water leaks out from tiny, thin-walled blood vessels and into our body. This leaked water can cause swelling in the soft tissues in the body. You may see puffy swelling in the legs and arms. As albumin levels go down, swelling worsens, often spreading from the legs all the way to the hips, arms, chest, and the stomach, as in Simon's case. Eventually the whole body may become puffy, and water may collect in the internal spaces, filling the abdominal cavity and causing a distended abdomen that is full of water. Water can fill the space between the layers of your lungs and cause difficulty breathing. When you see this kind of swelling, you need to understand that the liver failure has progressed significantly.

Bile is probably the most visible, most well-known substance the liver makes. It is also responsible for the most commonly known symptom of liver failure— jaundice. Bile is a pigmented compound. Produced inside the liver, its main function is to help digest fat. It collects into a system of small tubes inside the liver and comes out of a special collecting tube. This collecting tube takes bile into a sac called the gall bladder. The gall bladder stores the bile and releases it into the upper part of the intestine when needed. There is normally very little bile in blood because most bile is collected by the tubes.

The liver is a very resilient organ. It can suffer multiple assaults and instances of abuse and still repair itself. When you drink large amounts of alcohol for a few days, your liver is damaged. However, when you stop drinking, your liver works hard to repair the damage and usually bounces back within a few days. After steady abuse, your self-repair system becomes overwhelmed. That's why it takes years of severe abuse to cause permanent liver failure. Your liver still continues to repair the damage every day, but the process becomes less than perfect. The damaged liver cells continue to regenerate, but they fail to maintain the original smooth texture of the liver. They slowly start to accumulate scars from the repeated cycles of damage and repair. This scar tissue disrupts the delicate system of tubes that collect and drain bile. As a result, bile starts to leak into the blood. As the blood level of bile goes up, it stains your skin and other membranes, leaving your skin, eyes, and tongue with a yellowish hue. As the level goes higher, the discoloration becomes more pronounced, and you appear strikingly jaundiced.

Simon's liver failure did not show any signs of improvement. He was severely jaundiced. His skin and eyes had a distinctly yellow discoloration due to high levels of bile in his blood. Bile is a by-product of our red blood cells. In a normal person, red blood cells are constantly being made and destroyed to ensure a constant supply of young and healthy cells capable of supplying oxygen to the whole body. Your red blood cells live an average of about three months. When they die, they produce a pigment called bile. It is the final by-product of dead red blood cells. Your liver picks up those pigments from the blood and converts them into a chemically different form, releasing them into the upper part of your intestine, where they work as part of the digestive juices that digest the fat in food. When the liver is damaged, bile pigments from the blood are not collected properly and begin to back up and accumulate in the blood. These unconverted pigments cause the skin and eyes to appear yellowish and sickly—jaundiced.

The liver is also the main organ that processes nutrition in your food. To enable the liver to do this efficiently, your body has developed a special set of veins, called portal veins, which are abundant in the GI tract. When your GI tract absorbs nutrition from digested food and dissolves it in your blood, this nutrient-rich blood is transported to your portal veins. Before going to the rest of the body, these portal veins lead directly to the liver. The nutrient-rich blood goes inside the liver for processing before being released into the rest of the body. Inside the liver, these blood vessels branch out into tiny vessels that distribute the blood for efficient processing. These branches then slowly combine to form larger branches, eventually leading to a normal-sized vein that goes out of the liver and feeds this blood into regular veins.

When the liver is scarred from years of continuous abuse, this sophisticated system of specialized blood flow is disrupted, leading to backward blood flow and increased pressure on the veins close to the GI tract. When the veins become distended and swollen, they are called varicose veins, and they are very susceptible to erosion. Varicose veins in the food pipe are especially prone to tearing and rupturing. When they do, blood gushes out of them because of increased pressure. The resulting bleeding can be immediately life threatening. You may bleed to death within a few hours. If doctors had not quickly found the source of Simon's bleeding, he would have died that same day.

We will revisit liver failure in chapter 13.

11. Just a Small Heart Attack

How a "Small" Heart Attack Didn't Feel So Small to Laura

When the diagnosis you get doesn't seem to fit, don't stop looking for a better one.

Laura had been healthy for as long as she could remember. At thirty-five, she was physically active, and her days were usually busy. Taking care of her two children, ages three and five, was a handful. She had no health problems—her only hospital visits had been for the births of her children—and she wasn't on any medication except for birth control.

That morning Laura rose at nine and made breakfast for herself and for her kids. Her husband was out of town for a business meeting. When she got up to collect the dishes, she suddenly felt very light-headed. A sharp, stabbing pain shot through the left side of her chest, almost directly above where she knew her heart must be. Worried she might collapse and faint, she sat down again very slowly. *This must be what a heart attack feels like*, she thought weakly. She felt as though she had lost all the energy in her body in an instant. With what strength she had left, she dialed 911 and said she might be having a heart attack. After trying her husband's cell phone and only reaching his voice mail, Laura closed her eyes and tried to relax, despite her children peppering her with questions. When the paramedics arrived, Laura asked if one of them could go around to her neighbor's and see if she would keep an eye on the kids. After her neighbor took the kids, the paramedics asked Laura about her condition. Was she still having chest pain?

"Yes, it still hurts, right here, just above my heart." Laura weakly tapped where her chest hurt.

The paramedics lifted her onto a stretcher and checked her vitals. They noted she had a temperature of 97.8 degrees, a heart rate of 100 beats per minute, a respiratory rate of 20 breaths per minute, and a blood pressure of 98/46 milliliters of mercury. They gave her a nitroglycerin pill to put under her tongue and took her to the hospital in the ambulance.

On the way, the paramedics were able to perform an EKG. It showed sinus tachycardia (a normal heart rhythm with a faster than normal rate) but was otherwise normal. They gave her some oxygen and sent the EKG to the ER. By the time they arrived, Laura's chest pain had lessened but was still bothering her. She was still feeling very weak. When she tried to lift her head, she thought she might faint. After another EKG, Laura met with a doctor, who had examined the two EKGs side by side.

"What were you doing when the pain started?" the doctor asked. "Where did you feel it?"

"Well," Laura said carefully, "it started all of a sudden right when I got up from the breakfast table. I felt it right above my heart—in the middle of my chest but slightly to the left." She pointed to the left side of her chest. "Right above my heart," she repeated. "Isn't that where the heart is?"

"Yes, it is, but did you feel the pain go anywhere or did it just stay put?"

"It kind of stayed there, right there. It's still there, but the shot seems to have taken the edge off."

"Did you have any trouble breathing with the chest pain?"

"No." Laura shook her head. "No, I didn't. But taking deep breaths made the pain worse. The pain is like something heavy and sharp cutting into my heart. It made me feel weak instantly. I didn't have trouble breathing, but it was incredibly painful and took a lot of effort—I broke out into a sweat."

"Well," the doctor said after a pause, "so far the EKG only shows that your heart is running a little faster than normal, but there are no signs of major heart attack. We'll have to wait for the blood tests to see if you had a minor heart attack or something else. I'll have the nurse watch you closely until we get the test results back. In the meantime, I want to watch your blood pressure closely to make sure it doesn't get any lower as well as keep an eye on your heart rhythm to check for any abnormality. When the blood tests come back in about twenty to thirty minutes, we'll chat again."

Laura waited anxiously. The nurse gave her one more shot of morphine to dull the pain and help her rest. She told Laura that her heart rate was getting better but that her blood pressure was still borderline low.

Thirty minutes started to feel too long. How could she wait that long to find out if she'd had a heart attack? As she grew anxious again, her doctor returned with the results of her blood tests, which indicated that Laura might have had a small heart attack. Her troponin levels were slightly higher than normal, which is often a sign of a heart attack. A low positive troponin level usually suggested a minor heart attack or a heart attack in progress, the doctor explained. He wanted to admit Laura to the hospital and keep her overnight. He also wanted to get some follow-up tests done the next morning and perform a cardiac cath.

"A cardiac what?" Laura asked.

"I'm sorry—a cardiac catheter," the doctor clarified. "The heart doctor will give you more details, but a cardiac cath is a procedure. The doctor inserts a small catheter inside your artery, usually from your groin area, and guides it all the way into your heart to examine the arteries that supply blood to your heart muscles. They may also open blockages and put stents in depending on what they find."

Laura agreed to stay overnight, even though she just wanted to go home to her kids. After she had settled into her room, the admitting doctor came in to examine her. He asked her all the same questions that the ER doctor asked, but Laura was too anxious after hearing about the possibility of a heart attack. She couldn't bear the thought of another round of precautionary diagnostic questions. She interrupted the doctor.

"I'm sorry, Doctor, but before we go any further, I just want to say that the other doctor told me I may have had a small or minor heart attack. But small doesn't describe the pain I felt. The moment I stood up in the kitchen, I knew something was terribly wrong. In an instant, I felt drained of all my energy. All of it. It didn't feel minor. Does it sound minor to you?"

The doctor looked at Laura and nodded slowly.

"Thank you for telling me that, Laura. I've been wondering myself if there might be another possible cause of your chest pain. I'd like to go ahead and get a CAT scan of your chest to rule out any other event or failure."

"But, Doctor," Laura pleaded, "if it's not a heart attack, then what is it?"

"I can't rule out a heart attack, Laura. However, based on the description of your symptoms, I think it might be a better idea to look for other problems before we confirm the diagnosis of a heart attack. The CAT scan will look at your lungs and the blood vessels in your chest. I want to make sure there are no blood clots in your lungs or problems with your major chest arteries. I'll order it immediately, and I'll be back as soon as the results are in. I'll see you soon."

With that, the doctor left. Radiology technicians arrived and took Laura down for the CAT scan. They checked her IV line, flushing it to make sure it worked.

Then they hung a small bag of iodine-based contrast material on her IV pole and connected it to the IV line in her arm. They explained that the dye would flow into her blood and light the scanned images. It would help them better visualize her blood vessels and enhance the overall contrast of the x-ray images. The whole test would only take about ten minutes.

They were right. Ten minutes later, Laura was back in her room. Twenty minutes after that, the doctor reappeared with the CAT scan result and a tight frown on his face.

"What's wrong?" Laura asked. She didn't like the look on her doctor's face.

"Laura," the doctor said, "it seems like you had a fairly large blood clot in your lungs."

"Is that worse than a heart attack?"

"Well...it's different. Let me see if I can explain it to you in here." The doctor went to the whiteboard on the far wall and sketched a diagram of the outside of the heart and the lungs. He drew a series of arrows to demonstrate the path of blood flow from the right side of the heart to the lungs and then back into the left side of the heart. Between the right side of the heart and the lungs, he scribbled a large, messy dot. "That's a clot," he said, pointing to the spot. "The clot is on a major branch of the artery that carries blood from the right side of your heart to your lungs. When this clot cut off the supply of blood to part of your lungs, you felt the pain. This clot also prevented blood from flowing out freely to your lungs from the right side of your heart. As a result, pressure on your heart caused strain to the thin-walled right side of your heart. That strain caused the same chemical usually released with heart attack to be released, which is why it looked like you had a minor heart attack."

"That's what made me so weak? It sounds serious."

Laura tried to wrap her head around the news.

"It is serious. It's not minor at all. You felt faint because the left side of your heart filled up with blood returning from your lungs. The blood clot in your lungs prevented the free flow of blood inside the blood vessels in your lungs, and the amount of blood returning to the left side of your heart dropped. The amount of blood available for pumping in the left side of your heart went down and could not effectively supply blood to the rest of your body. Your heart tried to compensate for this deficit by beating faster as the amount of blood pumped with each beat decreased. Your heart was barely able to maintain your blood pressure. That's why you felt very weak and almost fainted. When we infused saline into your veins, it temporarily increased the volume of your circulating blood, and your heart was able to pump out a little more blood. That's why you felt somewhat better. I think this blood clot explains all of your symptoms and also explains why you seemed like you'd had a minor heart attack at first glance."

"Doctor, I'm so relieved to know what's going on—but what happens next? Will I recover?"

"I'll start you on blood thinners."

"So they'll dissolve the clot and get blood flowing again?" Laura asked.

"Actually it won't dissolve the clot. It will just thin the blood enough to prevent further clots so the clot can't get bigger. Of course when I say 'thin,' I'm not referring to the actual density of your blood. I'm describing your blood's clotting ability. Blood that clots easily is called 'thick,' and blood that doesn't is called 'thin.' Over the next few weeks, maybe months, your body will work to slowly and naturally dissolve the clot by itself."

"Can't you just go in and take out the clot to clear the blockage just like they planned to do when they thought

I had a heart attack?"

The doctor shook his head.

"It's just not the same thing, Laura. It's more difficult to clear a blockage inside blood vessels in the lungs than it is to clear a blockage in the artery supplying blood to the heart muscles. While heart arteries are relatively easy to locate, blood vessels inside the lungs are not that easily accessible. Locating them requires a riskier and much more invasive procedure that's only done when the blood clot is life threatening. In your case, if your heart hadn't been able to pump enough blood to maintain a near-normal blood pressure, you could have collapsed. If your blood pressure had remained low, despite treatment, we would have considered taking you to the operating room to clear that clot. But things look like they're a little more stable now. You don't need the surgery. If things get worse, we may have to reconsider surgery as an option, but I think it isn't necessary at this point."

Laura asked what had caused the blood clot, but the doctor told her that it was impossible to determine the cause. There were many risk factors, the biggest of which was a family history. Fortunately this was Laura's first blood clot, and she had no family history.

A nurse gave Laura a shot of Lovenox, a blood thinner, under her skin. Lovenox, she explained, contained an active ingredient that combated a clotting protein. When the activity of this key, protein-based chemical went down, it lowered the blood's ability to clot. Lovenox was fast acting and useful in the short term. However, it was not normally considered appropriate for long-term use, as it was quite expensive and had to be injected right under the skin.

A longer-term option, the nurse told Laura, was Coumadin, a widely available, inexpensive blood thinner that reduced the amount of vitamin K in the body.

Vitamin K was one of the essential elements required by the liver to manufacture clotting factors. When vitamin-K levels went down, the level of clotting factors in the blood decreased and the blood became "thin." This made Coumadin more dangerous than Lovenox because it could reduce the body's vitamin-K levels drastically. If allowed to completely deplete the body's vitamin-K levels, Coumadin could cause a patient to bleed to death. When taking Coumadin, regular blood tests were always necessary to check the coagulability of the blood.

Laura thanked the nurse. When she was discharged from the hospital, she remained on Coumadin for six months.

Teaching Points

Basic Approach: Diagnostic Tests

Diagnostic tests used in medical practice are very helpful aids in making or rejecting diagnoses, but they can sometimes be very misleading. If a diagnostic test suggests one diagnosis, and your body is trying to lead you to a different diagnosis, it is important to listen to your body. You need to clearly communicate what your body is trying to tell you to your doctor. His or her focus cannot just be on the diagnostic results.

No matter how expensive or technologically advanced test equipment is, no single medical test can be 100 percent accurate in predicting the presence or absence of a disease. There will always be some patients who test positive without having the disease. Conversely there will always be patients who test negative but do, in fact, have the disease.

Since all tests are imperfect, doctors usually like to know how imperfect a particular test is. To gauge accuracy, they look at two important factors: sensitivity and specificity. If a test is 90 percent sensitive, nine out of ten patients will correctly test positive. The tenth patient will falsely test negative. In actual practice, if a test has a sensitivity of 90 percent, it is considered a very sensitive test. This means that even a very sensitive test misses one out of ten diagnoses. The other factor doctors look at when evaluating a test is its specificity. Specificity refers to the percentage of patients who correctly test negative for a disease. A 90 percent specificity means that nine out of ten patients will test correctly negative, and one will test falsely positive. If doctors based their diagnoses solely on these tests, one in every ten patients might be misdiagnosed.

In Laura's case, doctors were testing her blood to determine her troponin level. Troponin levels test very sensitively for a heart attack and also very specifically, but the sensitivity is greater than specificity. No matter what number the test turns up, it will always indicate false positives and false negatives. As the specificity is lower, there will be more false positives than false negatives. In other words, some conditions will be labeled a heart attack based solely on test results.

As we saw in Laura's case, one false positive can be the difference between dying from a blood clot and catching it before it gets any worse. Based on the positive troponin, Laura's first doctor diagnosed her as having a small heart attack, even though her description of her symptoms didn't quite line up with a small heart attack. The kind of pain she described was actually closer to that of lung-lining irritation than to that of an aching heart muscle.

When your doctor gives you a diagnosis, do not accept it at face value. Ask what that diagnosis means. Then ask how that event inside your body might make you feel. If the diagnosis matches up with what you feel, then you can rest assured. If the diagnosis does not match what you feel, tell the doctor exactly what you are feeling and ask if it could be something else.

Organ System: The Lungs and Blood Clots

As you may recall from our discussion of the lungs in chapter 6, used blood from your body returns to the lungs in the exchange of oxygen and carbon dioxide. This used blood is collected by a low-pressure system of blood vessels called the veins. Veins are complex systems made up of tiny blood vessels, called capillaries. The capillaries facilitate the delivery of oxygen and nutrients to our tissues from the blood. Then they collect the used blood and combine to form larger blood vessels, which eventually form the veins. Smaller veins fuse together and form larger veins that return to the heart and then to the lungs. Inside the lungs, the veins divide again into smaller and smaller branches until they are thin enough to fit inside the air sacs. In the air sacs, they get oxygen and lose carbon dioxide. After that, they start to fuse again and finally return to the left heart to be pumped back to the body. Veins returning blood to the right side of the heart are thinly walled. The blood flowing through them flows slowly. If a clot forms in one of these veins, the clot can travel all the way to the right side of the heart and then to the lungs. In the lungs, these clots get trapped in dividing blood vessels. Once a clot is bigger than its blood vessel, it gets stuck and blocks the flow of the blood downstream. The most common place for this kind of clot to form is in the leg veins.

Clots form in the leg veins under conditions such as long periods of limited leg mobility, long periods of standing, and overall decreased mobility. These conditions can cause disruption of normal blood flow, increased clotting ability, and disruption of leg veins. All of these glitches can lead to blood pooling and the formation of clots. Disruption of veins from trauma, surgery, or inflammation can also put you at risk for venous leg clots.

Your blood has a natural tendency to clot when it detects any disruption in normal flow. Clotting is a defense mechanism that your body uses to protect you from bleeding to death from injuries such as cuts and lacerations. When your veins are cut, your blood detects the abnormal blood flow and abnormal vein surface, and it starts to clot. The clotting slows your bleeding and eventually helps stop it. Your blood's ability to clot on its own is known as its coagulability. Inflammation, smoking, certain medications, cancers, and genetic predispositions are common issues that may increase your blood's coagulability.

Of course, not having these clotting risk factors does not mean that you're not at risk for a blood clot. Sometimes the risk factor can only be identified in hindsight. When you have an abrupt unexplained swelling in your legs, tell your doctor that you are worried about a blood clot. You'll learn more about leg clots in chapter 14. When you have unexplained pain in your chest, ask your doctor if you could have a blood clot in your lungs.

But chest pain isn't the only sign of a lung blood clot. There are other symptoms that are more easily recognized when you understand the clotting process that can occur in your lungs. As you know, a clot blocks the supply of blood downstream from the branch of the blood vessel it lodges on. So what happens to the blood?

Pressure builds up in the blood vessels as blood flow is obstructed. The blood begins to back up and flow in reverse. If the clot is blocking a main branch, blood flowing out of the right side of the heart may put so much pressure on the heart muscles that it may fail abruptly, and your blood circulation may collapse. This type of blood clot has been identified in people with

116

unexplained sudden-death syndrome. In other cases, the reduction in blood flow may not be bad enough to cause death but may cause fainting. Some people only get light-headed or dizzy instead of passing out. In most cases involving this type of blood clot, the heart beats faster to try to compensate for the reduced blood circulation.

A blood clot in the lungs also reduces the amount of oxygen in your blood. The oxygen inside the air sacks with the obstructed blood goes to waste, and your body doesn't receive enough oxygen. Sometimes shortness of breath may be the only sign that you have a blood clot in your lungs. The pain only happens when the clot somehow disrupts the lining of the lungs. Light-headedness or fainting only occurs when the disruption of blood circulation is severe enough.

No matter what symptoms you experience as the result of a blood clot in your lungs, there is one fact you need to be aware of: Symptoms of blood clots develop quickly. When that clot lodges into a branch of the blood vessel in your neck, it does so abruptly. When your symptoms begin abruptly, you need to make sure that your doctor considers the possibility of a blood clot or, as mentioned in chapter 1, a "vascular event."

12. Just a Little Blood

How Bob's Detectible Bleeding Was Just the Tip of the Iceberg

Sometimes symptoms that appear on the surface are just the tip of an iceberg. You must look deeper to understand the real problem.

At twenty-six years old, Bob was doing well for himself. He had his own landscaping business. New projects were coming in. He'd just traded in his old work truck for a newer model, and he'd hired two new workers as the business expanded. Bob was glad for the help and for the fact that he could afford it, especially since the workers required training. Training was never easy and usually came at a price—mistakes were bound to happen along the way. What Bob didn't know was that it would cost him more than time and money.

One day, he and one of the new hires were laying heavy stones on the ground. As he held one end of a particularly heavy slab, his helper tripped on a chain and lost his balance. The stone slipped, and Bob had to duck quickly out of the way, jerking his shoulder quite violently to avoid being hit. After a quick break, Bob and his team kept working without any other accidents that day.

Over the next few days, Bob developed a nagging pain in his right shoulder. A week later he went to the doctor, who took x-rays and found nothing. He prescribed Bob some pain pills and told him he could go home.

The next day, the pain was worse after the pain medication wore off. Bob went back to the doctor again and had an MRI done. The MRI revealed a minor

118

ligament strain—a partial tear from the injury with the joint still intact. He gave Bob prescription-strength Ibuprofen and told him that it might take a few weeks for the strain to heal completely.

At home, Bob found that the Ibuprofen worked nicely. The pain faded, and he was soon back in the field finishing his project, taking his eight hundred milligram pills four times a day. But after taking his pills on the evening of the fourth day, he felt a little nauseous when he went to bed. In the morning, he woke up feeling very weak. Walking to the bathroom, he felt oddly light-headed. After a bowel movement, he noticed dark-colored blood in his stool. At first, it was mixed with stool, but then it was followed by a large pool of a black, tarry substance that smelled distinctly like blood. Bob thought it was very strange, but he wasn't in pain. He headed into the living room, feeling exhausted and confused. He was thirsty, and his mouth was incredibly dry, but the thought of drinking water made him sick. He called the doctor's office. Something just wasn't right.

A nurse picked up the phone right away. After listening to Bob's symptoms, she suggested he head to the emergency room. He could be bleeding internally. He'd heard about how dangerous internal bleeding could be, so he called 911. Paramedics arrived shortly and checked his vitals. Noticing Bob's heart was beating a bit faster than normal, they took him to the nearest ER.

At the ER, Bob was seen fairly quickly once he described the black, tarry stool and said he was worried about internal bleeding. The nurse checked his vitals herself and found that his temperature was 97.6, his heart rate was 115, his blood pressure was 98/46, and he was breathing twenty times per minute. The nurse started an IV line while the doctor ordered some blood tests.

After the nurse drew four vials of blood in four

different color-coded tubes, the doctor entered as Bob examined the two IV lines in each of his arms, each infusing his veins with a saline solution. After introducing himself, he asked Bob what had happened.

"This morning—when I went to the bathroom—I found blood. Am I really bleeding internally?" Bob was getting more and more anxious by the minute.

"Well, I will find out as soon as I can. First let me ask you a few more questions to gather a few details. Did you have any pain in your abdomen when you woke up in the morning?"

Bob shook his head. "No."

"Did you feel any different or unusual?" the doctor asked.

"Yes," Bob said, nodding. "I was very weak. In fact, I think I got a little light-headed as I was walking to the bathroom."

"OK, now tell me what happened next," the doctor pressed.

"Well, I sat down on the toilet and started having a bowel movement. I looked down because it smelled different." He described how terrible it smelled, like burning blood. Afterward he was exhausted and had a terribly dry mouth. He had tried to drink some water, he explained, but that only made him feel nauseous. "That's when I knew something was off. I called my doctor's office…and now I'm here."

The doctor made a note. "Have you ever had anything like this in the past?"

"No. Never."

"And did you feel this way last night before you went to bed?"

"No, I didn't."

"Did you have any pain, discomfort or anything like that in your stomach in the last few days?"

"No—" Bob stopped himself and thought. "Well,

now that you mention it, I think I felt a little sick to my stomach last night. It felt like a slight burning, almost like heartburn. I drank some water, and I felt better. I fell asleep right away."

"Have you had any other medical problems in the past?"

"Nothing serious. I had a little shoulder sprain on the job, but it feels better now. The prescription pain pills worked great, but—"

"Prescription pain pills?" the doctor interrupted Bob. "What prescription medication were you given?"

"Well, it was just ibuprofen, but it was the high-dose, prescription-strength one. It worked a whole lot better than the Advil I picked up at the store."

"How long have you been taking the high-dose ibuprofen?" the doctor asked, looking concerned.

"Less than a week, but I'm already running out. I'd say I've been taking it at least three times a day."

"A high dosage three times a day? Do you normally take that much ibuprofen?" The doctor looked more concerned now.

"No, not until this week."

The doctor examined Bob quickly and sent a sample of his stool out for testing. Bob asked again if he was bleeding internally. The doctor said it was certainly possible. Such a high, frequent dose of ibuprofen could cause stomach bleeding. As he left the room, he paused. "I'm glad you came in, Bob, and I don't want you to worry. We'll find out what's going on with you, and we'll take care of it. We'll take care of you."

Despite those reassurances, Bob started worrying again as soon as the doctor left. It was a shock to hear that his pain pills could have landed him in the ER. He just hadn't known, but he didn't want to jump to any conclusions because the test results weren't back yet. As he waited, he noticed he felt a little weaker again. The nurse noted that his blood pressure was getting a little lower than before, running at 92/40. She called the doctor who was on his way back to Bob's room with the test results. The doctor told her to infuse one liter of saline solution into Bob's veins and to run it as fast as she could. Soon Bob began to feel better, and his pressure improved to 100/45. His heart was still running around 110 to 115.

The doctor finally came back in. "Well," he said, "I have most of the test results back."

"And?" Bob inquired anxiously.

"Everything seems to point to the possibility of bleeding in your stomach. I can't say exactly how much blood you lost, but I think there's enough evidence to admit you to the hospital based on your symptoms."

"What will you do? I've already lost the blood—do you transfuse some more?"

"No," the doctor said. "Not right now. At this time, your hemoglobin count is at ten."

"Ten what?" Bob asked.

"Your hemoglobin level gives you an estimate of the red, oxygen-carrying cells in your blood."

"OK, so it's like my blood count, right?"

"Yes, it is related to the red-blood-cell count in your blood. Normal for males is fourteen to eighteen, but you don't really need a blood transfusion unless it goes below eight."

"OK…so ten is all right?"

The doctor shook his head. "I'm afraid it's too early to tell. You may have lost more blood than the test can detect at this time, based on your symptoms. Your bleeding happened in your stomach, but it came out in your stool. You also felt weak, dizzy and light-headed. Your blood pressure was on the lower side. Your blood has to travel a long distance from your stomach to come out in your stool, so I think there is more blood sitting in your intestine, slowly moving down. You must have lost a significant amount of blood to lower your blood pressure, and your numbers will continue to go down. Later you'll probably need a transfusion. For now, we'll watch you closely. I've started you on a medicine to help prevent any further bleeding. This medicine will run continuously through your veins and will keep the acid level in your stomach low. The nurses will take you upstairs now and watch you closely. They will be checking your blood every four hours to see how much your hemoglobin drops. I've already told our blood bank to get at least two units of blood ready to be transfused. If the next blood level is lower, they will give you that blood transfusion immediately."

They moved Bob up to his new room. Sure enough, as the doctor predicted, Bob's next blood test showed his hemoglobin was down to 8.1. The doctor went ahead and gave him those two units of blood.

Bob felt better after the transfusion. His next hemoglobin count went up to 9.5, and it remained above 9 for the next twenty-four hours. Since the bleeding occurred in his stomach, a gastroenterologist was consulted. Withholding food and water, the gastroenterologist performed an endoscopy. Numbing Bob's throat, she passed a tube with a camera down from the mouth and into the stomach through the food pipe. She saw that the bleeding had stopped but found evidence of inflammation and a few spots that appeared to have recent bleeding. She took some biopsies of those sites and removed the camera.

"Well, it looks like the bleeding has stopped," the doctor reassured Bob. "I believe it was caused by the high-dose ibuprofen that you were taking. High-dose ibuprofen and other medicines in that class are known to cause stomach bleeding like this. You're going to have to hold off and heal for a bit. You're no good to your business if you're sick like this."

Bob thanked the doctor. He knew she was right. In order to get back to business, he needed to get well first.

Teaching Points

Basic Approach: How You Feel

Your body has a way of warning you when something dangerous is going on inside. As you have learned, when you see a threat in the outside world, your body reacts. Your heart rate goes up and you start to sweat. Although you cannot see life-threatening dangers lurking inside the body, your body still senses them and reacts in a way that is similar to fight or fight. When the threat is overwhelming, your body exhibits the same signs of defeat and collapse.

It doesn't matter what kind of disease starts the process—the things you feel when your body is overwhelmed are often the same no matter what. If you are able to recognize that your body is overwhelmed, you can seek help before it's too late. Like Bob, when you feel too weak to do anything, too overwhelmed to even walk, too light-headed to stand up, or too shaky to function normally, you need to consider the possibility that this could be a sign that your body is overwhelmed with serious illness.

Organ System: GI Tract

In chapter 9, you learned about the GI tract and stomach bleeding. Now you've encountered one prominent cause of stomach bleeding: NSAIDs, or Nonsteroidal Anti-Inflammatory Drugs, such as Advil, Naproxen and Aleve. NSAID medications get their name from their anti-inflammatory properties, similar to steroids.

You are probably aware of the fact that most medications have adverse effects. NSAIDs are no exception. They can destroy the protective lining of the stomach. As you saw in chapter 7, when the protective barrier in the stomach gets destroyed, stomach acid leaks in and starts destroying the tissue. In the process, the acid erodes the blood vessels, causing bleeding. Sometimes this blood comes out as you vomit blood. In these cases, people seek help relatively early, and the risk of decompensation is low.

Sometimes the blood slowly flows down to the intestines and keeps on going. You may not feel much pain in your stomach. After traveling a long distance for a long period of time, the blood shows up in your stool as black, digested blood. It is hard to estimate the amount of blood you've lost by just looking at how much blood came out in the stool. Only the general effects of blood loss and the resulting stress communicated by your body can warn you.

When you have a rapid upper GI bleed, it is important to remember that even your blood test can significantly underestimate the amount of blood you have lost. Normally you look to your hemoglobin level to see how much blood you have lost. Hemoglobin gives you an estimate of the concentration of red, oxygen-carrying cells in your blood. When you lose blood, your hemoglobin level goes down. However, when you rapidly lose blood from your stomach, your hemoglobin level may test falsely higher. When you lose blood rapidly, you lose both red cells and water. The water from outside your blood vessels slowly seeps in and increases blood volume. When this process is complete, the blood becomes diluted, and your concentration of hemoglobin goes down. When the bleeding is too fast, the concentration of hemoglobin in the remaining blood inside the blood vessels may not have had enough time to become diluted. In such situations, it is important to check hemoglobin levels every few hours to determine

125

the real damage. When hemoglobin levels appear normal but your body is feeling severely stressed, IV fluids can help increase the amount of water into your blood vessels. IV fluids restore your blood volume quickly, allowing your doctor to estimate the amount of blood lost more accurately.

Due to their availability and effectiveness, NSAIDS are used by a very large number of people. While the percentage of people with problems is low, we still see many people with serious adverse effects because of the sheer number of patients using these medications. Even when prescribed by your doctor, NSAIDS should be taken with care.

13. Failure to Live

How Hiding Critical Information from His Doctors Cost Tyler His Life

The choice to keep key diagnostic information to yourself can be the choice between living and dying.

The first time his wife noticed he didn't look well, Tyler brushed it off. His coloring was strange, and his eyes looked tired and hollow. It was nothing, he said. He just needed more sleep.

The next day, Tyler looked much worse. His skin and eyes had a yellowish hue. This time, his wife didn't let him brush it off. She took him to an urgent-care facility, where a doctor performed an exam and some blood tests. The doctor didn't like what he found during the exam. Tyler showed signs of severe liver dysfunction, which caused the yellowing of his skin and eyes. His condition was acute, and the doctor recommended that Tyler go to the hospital at once. Tyler reluctantly agreed.

By the time Tyler was admitted to the hospital, he was exhausted. After examining the blood-test results, a new doctor asked Tyler some questions, which he answered slowly and quietly. His wife couldn't tell if he was just tired or a bit wary of the doctor.

"So how long would you say you haven't been feeling well?" the doctor asked.

"I'm not sure," Tyler answered defensively. "I was just tired this morning," he added. "I just needed more sleep."

"OK," the doctor persisted, "but what about before this morning? How long have you felt that way?"

"I don't know...maybe three or four days? I just haven't gotten enough sleep, really."

"Did you have any pain in your abdomen?"

"No," Tyler answered flatly. "I don't know what this has to do with anything."

"How much alcohol do you drink, Tyler?"

"I don't drink alcohol," came Tyler's monotone reply.

"All right, what medications you are taking?"

The doctor's question hung in the air before Tyler replied, "I am not taking any medications."

The doctor continued his questions about Tyler's medical history. Tyler answered each question—about liver problems, past medical problems, blood transfusions—with a flat "no." A family history of liver problems? No. Recent travel outside the country? No. History of depression? No. Was Tyler currently depressed? No.

Finally the doctor finished his line of questioning and performed an examination. He listened to Tyler's chest and abdomen, pressing down on the abdomen to feel the liver and spleen. He checked Tyler's hands and feet for any swelling. He then instructed Tyler to hold out both of his arms and extend his wrists. The doctor gently pushed back on both of Tyler's outstretched hands and observed a flapping motion in both of his wrists. The doctor noted this finding carefully. Sighing, he explained that Tyler did appear to have liver damage but that he didn't know what caused it.

"The blood tests have shown that your liver is inflamed—it's not performing its tasks well. From the pattern of injury, I'm afraid that it could be caused by something acute and active. This damage is ongoing. If we can find the cause of the damage, we may be able to give you specific treatment. Usually the common causes are alcohol, drugs, toxins, and infection. But based on our conversation, it seems like you do not have any of those." The doctor looked closely at Tyler.

"That's right. I don't." Tyler avoided making eye contact.

"Are you absolutely sure about that?" the doctor persisted. "Maybe you took some herbal medicine or a diet supplement? A medicinal tea or painkiller? You may not even have regarded it as a medication."

Tyler shook his head. "No, I have not taken anything like that."

"OK, I'll order some special blood tests and monitor your liver function closely. If we don't get any answer from the blood tests, we'll have to do a liver biopsy. It's an invasive procedure—we insert a needle in your liver and take a small sample to examine under a microscope."

Tyler underwent an ultrasound exam of his liver, several blood tests, and constant blood-pressure checks throughout the day. He was hooked up to a heart monitor in his room, and his wife settled in to wait by his bed for news from the doctor. In the afternoon, the doctor returned with good and bad news. He had the results back from Tyler's numerous diagnostic tests. The good news was that Tyler tested negative for HIV and for several different viruses that could cause liver injury. The bad news was that the cause of Tyler's liver damage was still a mystery. As he spoke, he studied Tyler's impassive face. Lying in a hospital bed, hooked up to a heart monitor, Tyler didn't seem like he was listening, even though his condition was clearly serious.

But Tyler's wife was worriedly listening, and she had questions.

"So what does that mean? What do we do now?"

"We will watch him closely and see how things turn out. If the liver damage gets worse, we may have to consider a liver transplant to save your husband's life."

The damage did get worse that night. Tyler's skin discoloration darkened. He became nauseous and vomited several times. His blood pressure started to drop, and he felt dizzy and light-headed. His face looked puffy, and his legs started to swell. Nurses transferred him down to the ICU and contacted the liver-transplant team. They started doing blood work to qualify him for a liver transplant. As they struggled to keep his blood pressure up, the doctor took Tyler's wife aside. Tyler's condition was getting worse, he said. The transplant team was working very hard to find a suitable donor, but there was a chance that it might be too late by the time they found one. Tyler's wife gasped. Her eyes brimmed with tears, and she looked at her husband, who was too weak to show any emotion. He stared at the doctor silently.

As Tyler's blood pressure continued to drop, he began to have trouble breathing. A team of doctors intubated him and hooked him up to a ventilator. They continued to push fluids and medications through his veins, but his blood pressure continued to go down despite the three different medications that were now working to force his heart and his blood vessels to increase the blood pressure. The doctors increased dosages on all three medications to achieve the maximum effect. For a few minutes, the medicine seemed to increase Tyler's blood pressure. Then, all of a sudden, Tyler's pressure plummeted, and his pulse disappeared. The doctors called a code blue and started CPR to no avail. Although there was still some electrical activity in his heart, Tyler's pulse was gone. The doctors continued several cycles of CPR and medications, but they were unable to revive him. He was pronounced dead.

The reason for his liver failure was still a mystery. The doctor called the chaplain to comfort Tyler's wife and started the postmortem paperwork. Tyler's wife started going through her husband's belongings. As she did, she found an envelope in his jacket packet. She opened it and dropped it. It was a suicide note. Picking it up slowly, Tyler's wife read the note. It said that Tyler had been extremely depressed and had decided to end his life. Two weeks ago, he had taken one hundred Tylenol tabs without telling anyone. By the time his wife noticed that he was sick, the Tylenol had caused irreversible liver damage, but the drug in his blood had dropped to undetectable levels. The doctor watched the chaplain help Tyler's widow sit down. He shook his head. Life was still a mystery.

Teaching Points

Basic Approach: Holding Back Information

This sad story just shows how hard it is to reach the correct diagnosis when the patient is not honest with the doctor. Even with modern medical technology, diagnostic tests, and equipment, the doctor cannot always uncover the truth when the patient deliberately withholds information. This is because medical tests cannot predict any diagnosis without background. The backstory tells the doctor what to look for in test results. A positive or negative test may have a different significance in different scenarios, just as you saw in chapter 7.

In chapter 7, the diagnosis of a stroke was made after the head CT was found to be negative. The diagnosis was based on the provided narrative and was confirmed by a test that did not show anything abnormal. While it may sound strange that a normal test can point to the diagnosis of an abnormal condition, it can. And it did.

The same test can have totally different and sometimes contradictory meanings based on the reason for testing. In most situations, a normal head CT is reassuring. If the patient presents with a bad headache, a normal CT scan is good news.

If Tyler's doctor had known about the Tylenol overdose, the first blood test would have given him enough information to start treatment that could have saved Tyler's life. The negative Tylenol level would have simply been a confirmation of the fact that a few days had passed since the overdose. The elevated liver enzymes and bilirubin would have meant that the patient had ongoing, active liver failure from Tylenol overdose. He would not have lost precious time searching for the source of the liver failure.

Organ System: Liver Failure and Tylenol

While alcohol is one of the most common causes of long-term liver failure, Tylenol is one of the most common causes of rapid and short-term liver failure. In the Unites States, it is the most common cause of acute liver failure, both intentionally and unintentionally. Generally considered a very safe medication, Tylenol is easily available.

Many people who take Tylenol with the intention of overdosing change their minds and seek medical help afterward. If they go to the ER within a day or two of taking the pills, they can be treated with medicine that can prevent liver damage from happening. Many such patients are saved in emergency departments throughout the country. Sadly it appears that Tyler had done his research before he decided to end his life and deliberately misled his doctor.

People who overdose on Tylenol unintentionally may do so for a variety of reasons, but one particular reason is most common—narcotic pain addiction. Narcotic pain pills, such as Vicodin or Norco, combine an opioid (a type of narcotic) with Tylenol. Some people abuse these pills and use them as recreational drugs. They acquire the drugs illegally and start to take more and more pills.

They may develop a tolerance to the narcotic component of the pill over time. Meanwhile the Tylenol component eventually builds up to cause liver failure.

The symptoms of acute liver failure are somewhat different from those of the chronic liver failure you saw in chapter 7. A rapidly failing liver may dramatically change the body chemical makeup and can have drastic effects since the body does not have time to adapt to changes as with chronic liver failure.

When the liver fails rapidly, the processing of vital chemical reactions slows down or stops. As a result, the composition of chemicals flowing into the blood changes rapidly. Some of those chemicals can go to the brain and disrupt its normal function. They can make you confused, disoriented, irrational, or even agitated.

A rapidly failing liver may stop making proteins required to prevent water from leaking out of blood vessels. As a result, you can develop rapid swelling from the leakage. In addition to the swelling, the leakage can severely reduce the level of blood inside the veins. This reduced blood flow can cause problems in other vital organs in your body. The disruption of chemical composition of the body, along with the disruption of blood flow, can eventually lead to the failure of multiple organs. The lack of clotting factors can also cause excessive bleeding. All of these changes can be life threatening and, once liver failure has advanced, irreparable. The only treatment that may save your life in this situation is a liver transplant. However, the availability of donor livers is limited, and the window of opportunity when a patient is stable enough to undergo such an extensive procedure is very small.

14. Running Through My Veins

*How Donna Found Out the Hard Way about Venous
Blood Clots*

Learn about venous clots and how they are formed.

Donna was recovering from a complicated abdominal
surgery. She had a ruptured appendix and required an
open laparotomy, a surgical procedure that involves
cutting through the abdominal wall to gain access to the
abdominal cavity. Her recovery was slow. She was
weak, and the large wound in her abdomen resulting
from the surgery was still painful. She had also
developed an uncomfortable urinary tract infection that
had set in two days after her surgery. Her doctor had
prescribed an antibiotic. A mother of two, Donna was
relieved when her husband hired a nanny to help out
during her recovery. Her kids always came first. This
time, Donna needed to put herself first. If her two-year-
old or her four-year-old had been in pain following a
medical procedure, Donna would have followed up with
their doctor right away, but she didn't think to do that for
herself.

Now, three weeks after her surgery, Donna woke up
early on a Saturday morning and sensed that something
was wrong. When she got up to go to the bathroom, she
realized walking on her right foot was painful. Sitting
down, she bent to examine her leg more carefully, and
what she saw was frightening. Her right leg was
significantly swollen compared to her left leg. It had a
strong reddish hue and felt unnaturally warm to touch.
Worried, she went back into the bedroom and woke her
husband up. Looking at her leg, her husband's face
creased with worry. He convinced her to call the doctor
right away even though it was a Saturday.

Donna called her doctor's office and got an on-call nurse who was very concerned by Donna's symptoms. She advised Donna to have her husband take her straight to the ER. Her husband called the nanny and made sure the kids would be taken care of. As soon as the nanny arrived, he drove her to ER. After registration, a nurse took Donna to a private room in the ER to wait for a doctor. When the doctor arrived, he had many questions.

"When did this happen?" the doctor asked as he studied Donna's leg.

"I don't really know," Donna said. "I mean, my legs looked normal when I went to bed last night. I woke up like this."

"Did you have any pain in your legs before you went to bed? What about fevers or chills?"

"No fevers or chills, but I have had some leg cramps now and then since my surgery. I don't remember having them last night, though."

"Are you able to walk?" he asked.

"Yes," Donna said, "I can walk on it, but it hurts a lot."

"How would you describe your pain?" The doctor waited.

"Well," Donna said slowly, trying to describe her pain as accurately as possible, "it feels like a throbbing pressure. It gets worse whenever I try to stand or walk. When I stand on my leg, the pain gets really sharp."

"And where exactly do you feel your pain?"

"It's strongest in my calf, but it shoots up the back of my thigh when I stand or walk." She waited as the doctor wrote something down.

"On a scale of one to ten, how would you rate your pain?"

"When I am lying down and not moving, I'd say it's at a three or a four. When I walk? When I walk, it's an eight or a nine."

"Has anything like this happened before, Donna?"

"No." Donna shook her head.

"Now I see that you had surgery recently. Can you tell me what happened?"

"Well, I had this pain in my stomach for quite a while, but I was so busy with my kids that I kept ignoring it. One day, it got very intense, and I suddenly had a fever. I took Tylenol and ibuprofen, both of which seemed to help. My fever went away, so I decided to focus on my kids instead of going to the doctor. But the pain and fever kept coming back, so each time, I'd take the Tylenol and ibuprofen again. After a week of that cycle, the pain medicines didn't help anymore. My fever got much worse, and I started getting chills and hot flashes. I was exhausted and almost fainted. When I told my husband, he took me here, to the ER. My CAT scan showed that I was very sick and needed surgery right away. They kept me in the ICU for two days after the surgery because my blood pressure was very low, and the surgery was complicated. After that, I developed a urine infection and had to stay four more days before I was released to go home."

"Do you still have any pain in your abdomen now?"

"Not like the pain I had before, but my incision wound still hurts a little bit, especially when it gets stretched. It stretches when I walk. Now I only walk when I have to. I've actually been in bed most of the time since the surgery."

The doctor made a note. He asked whether Donna had had past issues with blood clots, which she hadn't, nor, his questions revealed, had she had any past medical problems aside from the recent surgery and urine infection—no shortness of breath or chest pain, no nausea or vomiting, and no dizziness or light-headedness. Noting all of Donna's responses, the doctor commenced a physical exam. He listened to her heart and lungs, looking at the surgical scar on her abdomen and pressing on her stomach to see if it was tender. He turned his attention to her legs, comparing the swollen right leg with the left. Touching the swollen area gently, the doctor felt excess warmth. He checked Donna's pulse on each foot. He could feel a normal, regular pulse in both legs.

"Well," the doctor said finally, "here's what I think. I think we need to make sure you don't have a blood clot in this leg. You had a recent surgery, you have not been walking much since the surgery, and you have this red, swollen, and painful leg. The likelihood of a blood clot is very high. I'm going to order an ultrasound of your leg right away as well as some routine blood tests. When I have the test results, I'll come back. In the meantime, I'll have the nurse give you a shot of morphine to get your pain under control."

"Thank you, Doctor," Donna said. She was relieved. The morphine shot made her feel better; the throbbing was gone. It also helped her get through the ultrasound exam.

The doctor came back in after about twenty minutes. "Well, it looks like you do have blood clots in your deep veins. It seems like there's one large clot running from slightly below your knee to your midthigh. I think it may be helpful to keep you overnight in the hospital for observation so we can start you on the blood thinners and make plans for long-term treatment, which may take up to six months."

Donna was taken upstairs for an EKG and a chest x-ray. A nurse hooked her up to a heart monitor. Another nurse fit her with a finger probe to continuously check her oxygen saturation.

A new doctor came in and started asking the same kinds of questions the ER doctor had asked. Donna waited until after the physical exam to ask about the blood clots.

"So, Doctor, what do you think caused the blood clot in my leg?"

"Well, blood clots can be caused by several factors. You had a recent surgery. During and after surgery, your blood-clotting system becomes more active as it attempts to prevent bleeding. You also had an infection with sepsis. Sepsis also increases the risk of blood clots. Last but not least, you remained in bed for most of your recovery because you were weak and in pain. That probably caused blood to pool in your legs. This combination of blood pooling and increased coagulability is probably what enabled the formation of clots in your leg veins."

The doctor explained that he would be prescribing Donna two different types of blood thinners. The important thing to remember would be that these blood thinners, unlike those prescribed for heart attacks and strokes, would only make her blood less likely to clot any further. They wouldn't actually dissolve the clot, like clot-busting medicines. The body would naturally and slowly dissolve the clot. However, the blood clot could attract more of the clotting factors and platelets, creating more clots, or the initial clot might grow larger. Often there was some sort of struggle between the clot-dissolving factors and clot-forming factors after blood-clot formation. Despite the risks, blood thinners would give the clot-dissolving factors a fighting chance to continue to slowly dissolve the clot without the danger of new clots.

Of the two blood thinners, the first one would be an injection. The second one would be a pill. The main difference between the injection and the pill was the onset of action. The injection directly suppressed one of the clotting factors, and the coagulability decreased rapidly. The pill, on the other hand, slowly depleted the basic ingredient needed to make the clotting factors and took some time to work.

"Since you'll need to inject yourself at home, a nurse will be here shortly to show you how to give yourself the shot. I know it sounds scary," the doctor said, "but it is relatively easy. Have you ever heard about or seen patients with diabetes giving themselves insulin shots?"

"Oh, yes, my grandma had diabetes, and she took her own insulin."

"Yes, the blood-thinner injection is similar to that. I will tell the nurse to make sure you practice here so that you're ready to do it at home. We have syringes filled with saline so that you can practice multiple times. The pills are a different story. Coumadin depletes your body's vitamin-K levels. Vitamin K is an essential element needed to make clotting factors. It may take anywhere between a few days and two weeks to deplete the vitamin K stored in your body. You need to keep injecting yourself until your blood is thin enough. You will need to go to the lab about every two days to get your blood checked for the right amount of thinness using an INR test. The test needs to read within two to three units to ensure the right amount of blood thinning. If it's less than two units, you need to keep doing the injections. If it gets higher than three, your doctor will call you to adjust the dose of your Coumadin. I have every confidence that you'll be comfortable with this routine in no time. It's not easy, but it's habitual."

Donna thanked the doctor. She knew these injections would be difficult to get used to, but she also knew it was time to start taking care of herself.

Teaching Points

Basic Approach: Leg Swelling

Leg swelling can occur for several different reasons.

When you find that your legs are swollen, it's useful to focus on the details that can help your doctor diagnose the cause of the swelling.

If the swelling is present equally in both legs, it's most likely unrelated to the legs. A problem originating in the leg itself cannot manifest equally and similarly in both legs. Since the legs are the lowest parts of your body when you sit or stand, anything that causes water to leak out from the blood vessels into the surrounding tissue can cause swelling. A number of organ malfunctions, including heart, kidney, and liver, can change the dynamics of the blood vessels, resulting in water seeping out of veins into the tissue. If there are any changes in the body that cause water leakage from the veins, they occur in the legs first because the blood inside the leg veins has to travel against gravity to return to the heart.

If only one of your legs is swollen, it means that the problem is related directly to that leg. You need to think about what might have happened to the leg in question. It may have been caused by a fall, a collision, or even a bug bite or a cut. If you recall any such event, describe it to your doctor because it most likely holds the key to the diagnosis of your leg swelling.

If you cannot recall anything that may have caused the localized swelling in just one leg, you need to think about possible blood clots inside the veins of your leg. This is the most important and practical teaching point in this chapter. Be warned that you may not have any of the risk factors that Donna had and still have blood clots. Please do not think that your leg swelling may not be a blood clot just because you do not have any known risk factors for blood clots. Many times, the risk factors are retrospectively discovered after your first blood clot.

Organ System: Leg Veins

The flow of blood in the deep veins of your legs is very slow and sluggish. Veins carry the used-up, low-oxygen blood back to the heart. This blood does not have much pressure and mostly flows back passively. This presents a particular problem for the legs because the blood has to flow against gravity.

There are certain things that help achieve this difficult goal. First, most large veins have valves in them. When blood climbs up these valves, it cannot return back to the lower leg because of these one-way valves, leaving the blood with no other path than to flow toward the heart. The leg muscles also help push the blood up toward the heart. When we move our legs, the leg muscles contract and relax, putting rhythmic pressure on the veins. They get squeezed and the blood flows up. The valves ensure that the squeezing action helps move blood in the right direction. Any disruption in this mechanism can cause the blood to pool in the leg veins and can result in blood clots.

Anything that increases the coagulability of the blood can increase the risk of blood clots. Disruption in venous flow and increase in coagulability can increase the risk of blood clots even further. Donna had both.

15. The Clot Thickens

How Arthur's Arterial Clot Turned Catastrophic

Learn how arterial clots are different from venous clots and how they form.

Arthur was a smoker. There was nothing he loved more than a good cigarette. He'd been smoking a long time—ever since he was eighteen. He often went through several packs a day. Now, at sixty-five, he'd managed to get down to just one pack a day. Aside from a smoker's cough, Arthur seemed to have no health issues related to his smoking. He was fairly active and walked for at least thirty minutes every day. Despite his good health, he didn't like to go to the doctor. Doctors always told him he needed to quit smoking. On this morning, shortly after his birthday, he had not been to a doctor in the last ten years.

As he took his morning walk, Arthur felt more tired than usual. Turning around earlier than normal, he noticed that his left leg felt strange and then became genuinely painful. By the time he reached his house, he was practically limping. In his living room, he sat on the couch and took off his shoes and socks. He was shocked to see the state of his left foot.

His leg was incredibly pale with a bluish hue. It was cold and slightly numb to the touch. Worried, he called to his wife, who was in the kitchen.

"Honey, something's wrong with my leg!"

His wife came running in. "Oh my God, it looks horrible. Does it hurt? I think we should call my doctor."

She called her doctor's office but was told there weren't any openings for new patients until next week.

"You don't understand," Arthur's wife explained, "my husband's leg looks horrible. We can't wait until

142

next week."

The receptionist suggested that Arthur go to the ER. Arthur's wife thanked the receptionist and drove her husband to the ER. Once there, the nurse took one look at his leg and called the doctor. She arranged for Arthur to be moved to a private room right away.

The doctor came in and looked at Arthur's leg. He asked Arthur to tell him what happened and when he had first noticed something was wrong.

"Probably about half an hour ago?" Arthur approximated. "I was walking home from my daily walk, and my left leg started hurting. At first it was just an ache, but it kept getting worse, and I was almost limping by the time I got home. When I took my shoes off, this is how it looked."

"On your daily walks, did you ever have any leg pain like this before? Any aches or discomfort in your calf?"

"No, I would sometimes get a little tired if I went too far, but it never hurt like this."

"Have you had any heart attacks or strokes in the past?"

"Never," Arthur said.

The doctor then proceeded to examine Arthur quickly. He could not feel any pulse in the left leg. He grabbed a small, handheld Doppler unit to double-check Arthur's pulse but detected nothing.

"Well," the doctor said, shaking his head, "I think you have a clogged artery in your leg. This is a medical emergency. I will start you on a blood thinner right away and get a vascular surgeon on board as you may need urgent surgery."

"Doctor, what kind of surgery are we talking about?" Arthur was confused. This seemed to all come out of nowhere.

"Arthur, you may have plaque in your artery," the doctor explained. "Smoking is a major factor that can increase the risk of something like this. In any case, I detected no pulse in your left leg, which means your leg is not getting the blood it needs. If we do not restore blood flow quickly, your leg could be permanently damaged. A blood thinner will prevent the clot from getting bigger, but I think you may also need surgery to restore blood flow since a blood clot functions much like a heart attack. The vascular surgeon will decide the exact type of surgery, but it will most likely involve creating a bypass to supply blood to the organ affected by the clogged artery. As with a heart attack, time is invaluable, so I will start the blood thinner and call the surgeon right away."

The doctor started Arthur on an intravenous blood thinner called heparin. A quick acting medication that inhibits the natural clotting factors in the blood, heparin's effect needs to be monitored very closely to achieve the right level of blood thinning. Although it requires close observation, heparin has the advantage of working quickly and wearing off quickly.

Twenty minutes later, the vascular surgeon came in to examine Arthur.

"I think the best way to treat this is to take you to the operating room right away. That will give us the best chance to restore blood flow and save your leg. I will have the nurses shut the blood thinner off. Once the initial loading dose of heparin has worn off, we'll prepare the operating room. I'll try my best to restore the blood flow to your leg by bypassing this obstructed artery. This surgery has its risks, but it's our best shot at saving your leg."

"OK," Arthur said, worried, "if that's what I need."

Two hours after the surgery, Arthur woke up in a different hospital room. The surgery had been successful. He still had some pain in his leg, but he felt much better. His leg was no longer blue. Three days later, he was able to return home.

The hospital visit was a wake-up call for Arthur. He made a decision to quit smoking the day he was discharged. He also made sure that he went to the doctor for regular visits every three months after that.

Teaching Points

Basic Approach: Blocked Arteries

In the previous chapter, you learned about blood clots in leg veins. In this chapter, you encountered clogged leg arteries. The important difference between clots in your veins and clogged arteries is the effect each has on the blood supply. Blood clots in the veins do not cut off the supply of blood to any organ, while clogged arteries do. This is because veins are part of the body's drainage system, not its supply chain. Veins drain used-up blood away from organs. Clogged arteries lead to stoppage of blood supply to organs that need it.

Organ System: Leg Arteries

Your legs need a constant supply of fresh oxygen and nutrients to survive. Major arteries supply this oxygen in the form of oxygenated blood. They expand when the heart pumps blood out, and they contract to their original size when the heart relaxes to collect the returned blood. This constant expansion and contraction is what creates a pulse in your leg arteries.

Your arteries have evolved to withstand this constant pressure and the force of contraction. Elastic and thickly walled, they have an inner lining that is very smooth and uniform that helps the blood glide through the arteries without turbulence. Anything that affects the smoothness and elasticity of these blood vessels can cause problems in the arteries.

Smoking, high cholesterol, and high blood pressure

are examples of risk factors that disrupt these smooth linings. You can think of the lining as the coating of a nonstick cooking pan. It helps maintain the smooth surface and prevents food from sticking to the layer underneath. In the case of your arteries, the coating prevents blood from getting stuck to the arterial walls. When there is a disruption in this coating, blood cells and cholesterol adhere to it and initiate the formation of plaque. The plaque continues to grow as long as the risk factors for plaque formation persist. The arteries gradually narrow, resulting in the reduction of blood flow. Plaque can attract clotting factors and platelets, causing the formation of blood clots that drastically obstruct the flow of blood. These clots can also break off and clog the artery at a different site downstream from the initial site.

The process of plaque formation and the occlusion of blood flow is similar in arteries that supply blood to major body systems. The same risks that predispose someone to heart attack also predispose the same person to stroke, leg ischemia, and bowel ischemia. An ischemia is the term for a lack of blood or a loss of blood supply.

Sometimes the narrow arteries in the legs give off warning signs. When arteries become so narrow that blood flow is reduced but not completely obstructed, you may only experience symptoms with activity. When you are just resting, the reduced blood flow is enough to supply the oxygen and nutrients needed at rest. When you walk or run, however, your legs need more oxygen and more nutrients. Your muscles become more active and require more oxygen and nutrients. When the flow of blood is not enough to supply this increased demand, you experience pain in your legs. Usually this kind of pain is predictable. It comes on after a fixed amount of activity. It may come on after walking two blocks at a regular pace, but usually goes away promptly after a rest.

Unlike partial obstruction, complete and acute clogging of the artery can cause catastrophic changes that can result in complete loss of the affected leg. Timely intervention and surgery to reestablish the flow of blood can save your limb in such situations.

16. No Air

How Bret's Obesity Affected His Ability to Breathe

Learn what effect obesity can have on the heart and lungs and how it can lead to life-threatening complications.

Bret had struggled with his weight all his life. During college, he had been just a little overweight, but when he started his desk job as a software engineer, he kept putting on more pounds every year. Late nights and hours staring at a computer screen often left him too tired to exercise at the end of the day. He tried different diets but always ended up gaining the weight back, plus more. With every extra pound he gained, he became more and more tired until he was unable to do any exercise at all.

By Bret's thirty-eighth birthday, he weighed more than 380 pounds. He was tired all the time and every daily activity was exhausting. He drank cups and cups of coffee every day just to stay alert. Despite the strain, Bret was a hard worker. He took pride in the fact that he did good work and had earned several promotions. His office valued him and catered to his needs. He had a large, comfortable office chair. His desk and work space were modified to minimize movement and maximize productivity. Yes, he drank a lot of coffee, but he was happy and so was his company.

The year his oldest son started kindergarten, Bret finally decided he needed to do something about his weight. He started a walking program after work that involved gradually walking more and more every day. His goal was to be walking a mile daily by the end of the month.

It was very difficult in the beginning. The first day, he could hardly walk a block. He huffed and puffed, and his whole body ached. He kept trying to walk a little more every day, but he could never go more than two blocks without stopping to catch his breath. But Bret still persisted. He was committed to changing. After six months, though, he realized nothing was changing. He was still huffing and puffing after two blocks. He'd be exhausted and often unable to catch his breath. After having that same sensation for a few days, he decided that he would see a doctor before he tried the walking program again.

He took a day off from work and went to the doctor's office with his wife. The nurse took his height and weight and then started checking his vital signs. She put an oxygen probe on his finger to check his oxygen saturation. It only registered 79 percent. She checked on a different finger. It fluctuated between 78 and 81 percent but did not go higher than 82 percent no matter how many times she retested. She told him to take a few deep breaths but that did nothing to improve his oxygen-saturation level at all. She tried a different probe, thinking that one could be faulty, but it showed the same result. Just to be sure, she put that probe on her own finger, and it immediately registered 98 percent. The probe was working, but Bret's body was not. "Are you having any trouble breathing?" she asked, concerned. "Your oxygen level is too low."

Bret nodded. "Yes, I've been having some shortness of breath when I try to walk. That's why I'm here."

The nurse called the doctor, who looked at the oxygen monitor and asked, "Can you take a few deep breaths, Bret?"

Bret took a few breaths for the doctor, but his oxygen saturation remained low. The doctor asked the nurse to grab an oxygen tank. They started the flow of oxygen to

Bret's nose with a nasal cannula. They waited a few minutes and checked Bret's oxygen saturation again. It had slowly risen to 91 percent. The doctor listened to Bret's heart and his lungs.

"Well, your oxygen level was very low, Bret. It may have been running low for some time. We need to find out why and make appropriate treatment plans. I think the best way to do that will be to admit you to the hospital. The doctors there will be able to conduct more extensive investigations, watch you closely, and devise a treatment plan. If it's all right, I'll call the hospital and get you admitted there directly. I don't think you need to go through ER at this time."

Bret agreed and thanked the doctor. As the hospital was very close to the doctor's office, Bret's wife could drive her husband to the hospital herself. The doctor's staff helped Bret get situated in the passenger's seat with the oxygen tank.

At the admitting office, a nurse helped Bret into a wheelchair and secured the oxygen tank correctly next to him. After a quick registration process, she wheeled Bret up to his room on the third floor of the hospital. In his room, a new nurse checked Bret's vitals and obtained his basic medical history.

The doctor then came in the room. "I understand you're having trouble breathing," he said.

"Well, no, not at this time, but I was winded earlier when I moved a little too fast."

"Oh, I see." The doctor made a note. "How long have you felt that way?"

"Well, six months ago, I decided to try to lose some weight. I took up walking but always felt tired. It wasn't that bad, though, until now. In the last two weeks, I've begun to feel much worse. I feel like I have no energy, and walking a block or two can completely wind me."

"How much physical activity did you engage in

before you started walking?"

"Not much, I suppose. I'm a computer programmer, and I spend most of my time at my desk on my computer. My routine always ended with going home and watching TV until I fell asleep. I was so tired that I kept putting off exercise. Time just slowly went by. I know I'm overweight. That's why I tried to start walking, but now I know I can't do this on my own. That's why I'm here."

The doctor nodded. "Well, I'm glad that you're here. Do you get any chest pain or chest tightness when you walk?"

"No, I just run out of breath."

"Have you had any other medical problems in the past? Any history of heart attacks or blood clots in your family?"

"Aside from this shortness of breath, I've always felt fine. But I wouldn't know if I had something—I haven't really seen a doctor in years. And, no, no history of either blood clots or heart attacks in my family."

The doctor asked more questions—did Bret drink or smoke? Bret shook his head, and the doctor noted the answers on his chart. The doctor then listened to Bret's heart and lungs. He had some trouble listening through the extra weight but still detected no abnormal sounds in either Bret's heart or lungs.

"Well, from what you describe, Bret, it sounds like your oxygen levels are running very low. We'll need to do some tests to find out why. First off, I need to get a blood-gas analysis to find out the exact amount of oxygen and carbon dioxide in your blood. For this, we'll need an arterial blood sample, which comes from your arteries instead of your veins. I want it to be a room-air blood gas, though, so I'll be turning off the oxygen tank supply for a few minutes. I need to see how your blood-oxygen levels are without the support. Please tell me if you start to feel short of breath."

A nurse turned Bret's oxygen off. His oxygen saturation on the monitor slowly started to go down, settling, after a while, at 84 percent. The blood-gas technician drew an arterial blood sample effectively and sent it over to the lab for analysis. The nurse put Bret back on oxygen, and the doctor left to order a chest x-ray and some routine venal blood tests.

Once the doctor reviewed Bret's test results, he returned.

"Well, I have most of the test results here. The blood-gas analysis is the most important one. It seems like you have low oxygen and high carbon-dioxide content in your blood. Your bicarbonate level is also increased. It suggests that your breathing may have been inadequate for some time."

The doctor explained that the lungs drove oxygen into the blood and carbon dioxide out of the blood. Bret's lungs had not been very good at that.

"But—why?" Bret was confused. "Why would they do that?"

"Well, I can't say for certain yet, but the pattern of your symptoms and your blood-gas analysis suggests that the problem is due to a lack of ventilation. It means that your lungs are not moving enough for an effective gas exchange. They are not expanding and collapsing enough when you breathe in and out. Do you have any questions?"

Bret nodded. "What's the next step?

"Good question," the doctor said. "But I'm afraid the answer won't be clear without a few more tests. I'd like to order a CT scan of your chest. The CT scan will help me look at your lungs in more detail. It will also help me rule out blood clots or other problems in your lungs. The second test will be an ultrasound of your heart. It will tell me if you have any heart problems that may be associated with your shortness of breath. I'm afraid you're in for a busy afternoon."

The doctor was right. Bret had a very busy afternoon. First he had the CT scan. Technicians ran contrast material through his IV line while moving him back and forth on the CT scanner. When the scan was complete, they wheeled him back to his room, where an ECHO technician was already waiting to perform the heart ultrasound.

The technician put some jelly on the ECHO probe and moved the probe in different directions on Bret's chest, carefully looking at the images transmitted onto the machine screen. The probe, she explained, transmitted sound waves to the heart and detected the reflected sound wave coming off of the heart muscles. It also calculated the velocity and direction of blood flowing in and out of the different chambers of the heart.

Finally, in the late afternoon, Bret's doctor returned with the new test results. The CT scan had revealed that the lower section of each lung was slightly collapsed and wasn't expanding properly. Most likely the problem was secondary to the extra weight around Bret's abdomen. Otherwise the CT was normal—no blood clots or any other issues. The structure of the lungs appeared normal.

The sonogram was largely normal as well, with the exception of signs of increased pressure on the right side of the heart. The main reason for Bret's shortness of breath was obesity hypoventilation syndrome.

"I'm sorry," Bret said, stopping the doctor. "Hypoventi-what?"

"Obesity hypoventilation syndrome," the doctor repeated. "Or OHS. In the case of some patients who are overweight, the lungs have a hard time expanding. The air inside the lungs does not move enough to create an effective ventilation system. Without proper ventilation, your blood doesn't experience enough gas exchange to

153

move oxygen and carbon dioxide in and out of your blood. When your body goes through this for a long period of time, it tries to adjust to the low oxygen and high carbon-dioxide levels. The blood vessels in your lungs contract to try to squeeze a little more oxygen out of the small amount of air they have. When they do this for a long time, they can develop a high-pressure condition called pulmonary hypertension.

When the pressure inside the blood vessels of your lungs is high, the right side of your heart has to work extra hard to pump blood into the lungs. This pressure can eventually lead to heart failure. In your case, Bret, you just have a mild elevation of the pressure in the right side of your heart. Now there's a short-term solution and a long-term treatment plan for you to combat OHS."

"Wow." Bret shook his head. "Well, what's the short-term solution?"

"In the short term, this oxygen tank needs to go home with you. The extra oxygen will help relieve some of the pressure on the blood vessels in your lungs. Your body will also get some more oxygen and function better. The oxygen will, at the very least, halt the progression of your pulmonary hypertension."

"Oxygen? How long will I have to be on that?"

"Well, that's just the short-term solution, as I said. The long-term solution will address the root cause of the problem—your weight. Without working on your weight, we cannot work on your breathing problem. I'm glad you came in, Bret. I've seen obesity make so many people feel helpless and out of control. It's not easy to lose weight, but it is the only treatment, and it will improve your life quality exponentially in ways you never even expected. Any other treatment can only help you to a certain extent. I think it is best to work with your regular doctor, a dietician, and a physical therapist to create a balanced plan to achieve long-term weight control. If the plan fails, a gastric bypass may be another option to consider. It should be a last resort, though."

Bret nodded. "Of course. Surgery is the last thing I want. I'll try to lose this weight. Thanks for recommending a dietician and physical therapist. I realize now I can't do this on my own."

"Well, I am happy to hear that," the doctor said. "There's just one more thing I would like you to do—a sleep study at a sleep lab sometime in the next few weeks to monitor your breathing and oxygen levels while you sleep. Many patients with obesity hypoventilation syndrome also have some degree of obstructive sleep apnea. With obstructive sleep apnea, your air pipe collapses and becomes clogged as you sleep. It is important to see if you have that because we can treat it, improving your overall condition."

Bret thanked the doctor. His health had always come third for him—after his work and then after his family. But now he realized he had to put his health first to put his family first. He thought of his two sons.

"Doctor?" he asked.

"Yes?" the doctor stopped at the door.

"I have two young sons and…"

"You never want them to feel like this?" The doctor smiled sympathetically.

"That's right. How can I help them avoid this down the road? I never want them to feel like this."

"I'm sure your children are full of energy—encourage them to use it all. You can ask your physical therapist about this as well. Again, I'm glad you came in, Bret. I have faith that you can lose this weight."

Teaching Points

Basic Approach: Recognizing and Addressing Obesity Early

155

When your body is under stress, you know it. You may choose to ignore it, but it will eventually catch up with you. When you gain weight, you can feel the strain the excess weight puts on your body. When your weight reaches a certain point, you experience difficulty walking. Bending down to tie your shoes can feel impossible. Similarly, you feel the strain when you start to have trouble breathing. Many people feel it once the extra weight has already started to wear them down. Some of them realize and make changes to fight, while others give up and adjust their lifestyles to the new reality. Bret had gone down that second path, the one of least resistance. Now he would start the steeper climb up the path to changing his life.

Organ System: Ventilation in the Lungs

The inability to take deep breaths is a dangerous consequence of extreme obesity. Not everyone experiences it, and it's difficult to determine why that is. People who develop this condition experience a slow worsening of ventilation. As the ventilation grows progressively worse, the lungs become ineffective at blowing out carbon dioxide. The high carbon-dioxide levels cause increased acidity in the blood and trigger reactions to counteract the acid. These changes can increase weakness and fatigue.

The excess carbon dioxide begins to replace oxygen inside the small air sacs in your lungs. Eventually your lungs develop low oxygen levels, leading to the impairment of multiple vital organs, including your brain. Low oxygen levels can also trigger a series of changes that may result in heart and lung damage. When the blood vessels inside the air sacs sense an oxygen deficit, they try to squeeze the blood to absorb as much oxygen as possible. This action increases the oxygen levels temporarily, but it also increases the pressure inside these blood vessels. As the pressure continues to rise, it can impede the normal flow of blood from the right side of your heart to your lungs, eventually leading to heart failure. If treatment with oxygen is not started in time, these changes can be permanent. The blood vessels inside your lungs get used to the high blood pressure, and heart failure becomes irreversible. Blood eventually starts to flow backward. It backs out of the lungs into the right side of the heart and then back down to the major veins. The pressure inside your veins goes up, and water leaks out of small blood vessels. Eventually you develop severe swelling in both legs. In the end, there is not enough blood flow to the main circulation system. You run the risk of dying from heart failure and lack of oxygen.

17. Body Chemistry

How Harry Lost His Salt and Water—and Got Them Back

Learn the basic chemistry of salt and water and how it affects everything in your body.

Harry was your typical twenty-two-year-old college student. He had a roommate. He had finals. After finals, he went on spring break in Cancun.

It wasn't until he was on the way home from the airport that Harry knew something was wrong. He felt sick. He arrived home not a moment too soon, starting to vomit almost the moment he dropped his bags on the floor. After nearly not making it to the bathroom, he brought up a weekend's worth of salsa and chips, his main diet in Cancun. He continued to be sick for several hours, even after there was nothing left in his stomach. He felt weak and queasy. As he began to dry heave, severe cramps set in, as well as thin, watery diarrhea. Soon he was running to the bathroom almost every thirty minutes. When his nausea subsided, he started drinking water. It left a bad taste in his mouth, but he kept it down.

Exhausted, Harry fell asleep. He slept for an hour, but then the cramps set in again. He ran to the bathroom, and the diarrhea started again. He drank two glasses of water and went back to sleep. This cycle repeated all night long, and each time, he drank two glasses of water.

Toward morning, Harry's diarrhea slowed, and he slept for a few straight hours. When he woke up, his roommate was standing in the doorway, looking at him.

"Dude, are you OK?" his roommate asked. "You look really tired."

"Huh?" Harry asked weakly. He was exhausted. He

stared blearily at the wall, looking confused.

"Are you OK?"

"Um, yeah," Harry said. "Why? I'm just…really tired."

"I can see that," his roommate said, sitting down. "I guess you had a good time in Mexico?"

"Mexico?" Harry repeated hollowly. "What about Mexico?"

"How was—OK you're scaring me. What happened in Mexico?"

"Oh, well, I don't know. I don't remember. I just feel very tired. I think I just need to go back to sleep." Harry nodded to himself, and his eyelids drooped.

"OK, wow, you're really scaring me. I'm driving you to the hospital."

Harry nodded. In the car, he sat quietly as his roommate drove to the ER. He seemed to be in some kind of stupor. As they pulled up in the parking lot, Harry's roommate asked if he could walk on his own.

"I can walk," Harry said uncertainly, but after his roommate helped him out of the car, he found that he couldn't walk steadily.

"Wait here," his roommate said, shaking his head. "Just get back in the car. This isn't going to work."

Harry's roommate hurried into the ER. Seeing Harry so unsteady and unable to walk, as though he had been drinking, had shaken him. He spotted a nurse and approached her. "Excuse me, I drove my friend here because he looks very sick. I tried to get him out of the car, but he can't walk straight. I'm really worried. Can you ask someone to help me get him from the car?"

"I can help you," the nurse said. She got a wheelchair from behind the check-in desk and motioned to another nurse at the desk. "Where are you parked?"

"Right in the front. Thanks."

The two nurses ran out with him with the wheelchair.

They parked the wheelchair right next to the passenger-side door of the car and helped Harry get out of the car. All the while, Harry looked as though he was in a stupor.

Harry was taken to a hospital room and helped into bed. A new nurse started checking his vitals. His temperature was 97.6, pulse 110, respiration eighteen per minute, and his blood pressure was 110/45. His oxygen saturation was measured at 96 percent.

A doctor came in to talk to Harry. It wasn't easy. "Hello, Harry. Can you tell me when you started getting sick?"

"Don't know, really," came Harry's vacant reply.

"Do you know where you are, Harry?" the doctor asked, concerned.

"What? Yes...yes, I'm...here."

"Yes, Harry, but where are we?"

"Oh." Harry shook his head slowly, as though trying to clear it. "I don't know."

"Do you know what day it is?"

"Today? No. No, I'm not sure."

"And do you know who this person is?" the doctor asked, pointing to Harry's roommate.

"Yes, that's my roommate. Tim."

The doctor nodded, looking relieved. "Now are you having any pain anywhere?"

"No, not really, but I feel like I need to go to the bathroom. My stomach is cramping again."

"So have you been having constant diarrhea?" the doctor asked, concerned.

Harry nodded slowly.

"When did it start, Harry?" the doctor pressed.

"Well, I'm not sure." Harry gulped. "But I need to go again right now."

A nurse escorted Harry to the bathroom, and the doctor turned his attention to Tim. "When did he start acting like this?"

"I'm not sure. I know Harry went to Mexico for a weekend over spring break. It was his first time—I remember because he was so excited. He got home last night, but I only just came back this morning from visiting my parents. When I walked in the door, there he was. The whole place reeked—I think he'd been vomiting all night. It was all over the bathroom. He could barely focus on anything, so I brought him here. Is he going to be OK? Does he have food poisoning? I'd call his parents, but they're out of the country. Is there anything I can do? I've known Harry forever."

"Thanks, Tim. Do you know if he has any health issues? What about drug use or alcohol consumption?"

"No, we go way back. He's always been incredibly healthy. And he's never used drugs as far as I know. He's never been a smoker either. He has a beer or two once in a while."

The doctor thanked Tim and ordered a head CT scan, a chest x-ray, some routine blood tests, and a urine analysis. The head CT came back normal, as did the chest x-ray. The urine analysis showed only that his urine was too concentrated. Routine blood tests revealed the main problem.

Harry's blood chemistry was grossly abnormal. The level of sodium in his blood was very low at 121, as opposed to the normal level of 135. The level of potassium in his blood was also low at 2.9, with the normal level being 4. His urea-nitrogen level was elevated at forty-five, with the normal level being less than twenty. His creatinine level was mildly elevated at 1.5, as opposed to a normal 1.2.

The ER doctor decided that Harry needed to be hospitalized to correct the abnormal blood chemistry. He was confident that the abnormal blood chemistry had caused Harry's confusion.

Harry was transported to the ICU and monitored

closely. After examining Harry, the ICU doctor ordered IV fluids. He wanted to slowly correct Harry's blood sodium and potassium levels. He ordered blood chemistry work every four hours and adjusted the IV infusion based on the results. The next morning, Harry woke up, no longer confused and realized that he was in the hospital. When the doctor came in for morning rounds, he was pleased with Harry's condition.

"Well, you look much better this morning, Harry. How are you feeling now?" the ICU doctor asked.

"Thank you. I feel much better. But can you tell me what happened? I don't remember much from last night. I remember I was very sick when I came back from Mexico. I thought I just had some food poisoning. I kept vomiting and then the diarrhea started. I was getting very tired and thirsty. I was drinking plenty of water...and then...and then I don't really know what happened in the morning. I don't remember how I got here."

"Well, that makes perfect sense. I agree, you did have some kind of food poisoning, and that seems to have resolved by now. I think the reason why you were so tired and confused was because of dehydration caused by the food poisoning. The dehydration caused a very serious salt and water imbalance in your body."

"Wow, I didn't know that could happen. How?"

"You were vomiting and having diarrhea. You were losing water and electrolytes from both ends, quite literally. Electrolytes are basically mineral salts dissolved in your blood, such as sodium chloride, which is known as common table salt. The correct balance of this salt is vital to normal body and brain function. When the concentration of sodium in your body goes up or down, it can have a significant and devastating effect on the body. Your sodium concentration was incredibly low. It seems you replaced the water you lost when you were sick but not the sodium."

"That makes sense," Harry said, nodding. "Every time I got sick, I drank two big glasses of water. I didn't want to get dehydrated."

"Well, you had the right instinct," the doctor said. "That explains why your sodium level kept going down. When it reached a certain level, your brain could not function normally, and you became very confused."

"Wow, I didn't know salt was that important for my brain and body. I thought salt was a bad thing. I thought we needed to stay away from salt to become healthy. Was I wrong?"

The doctor explained that salt was actually very important, but that the balance between salt and water was even more important. The balance of salt and water was the basic factor that controlled pressure in the body. With the addition of too much salt, the blood would draw in more water to balance out the equilibrium, leading to higher blood pressure. With too little salt, water would leak out of the blood vessels to match salt deficiencies, leading to problems such as brain swelling and confusion, as in Harry's case.

Harry's sodium level eventually returned to normal. He felt much better and was able eat and drink normally without any nausea and vomiting. Soon his roommate returned to pick him up. All in all, this spring break had been a little too exciting.

Teaching Points

Basic Approach: Salt and Water

Most of your body fluids contain salt and water. Whenever you have a condition that takes away or wastes your body fluid, you need to think about salt and water imbalance. Excessive loss of body fluids can occur in many different situations. For instance, if it is too hot outside, and you don't drink enough water, you can lose salt and water through the evaporation of your sweat. If you have food poisoning, like Harry, or a stomach bug, you can lose salt and water when you vomit digestive fluids. If you are having liquid diarrhea, you can lose salt and water through your stool. If you have a condition that causes excessive urination, such as diabetes, this excess urine can carry away too much salt and water.

It is important to note that not all salt-water imbalances are caused by loss of salt and water. Sometimes consuming too much salt or too much water can cause a severe imbalance.

Organ System: Kidneys and the Balance Between Salt and Water

Drinking too much water can kill you. It may be difficult to imagine, but it's true. Little known but extremely dangerous, water poisoning can lead to death. Your blood requires a certain proportion of salt and water to function properly and to maintain your organs. Drinking water dilutes your blood and signals your kidneys to adjust the concentration of salt in your urine to get rid of excess water. Similarly, when you lose water or eat more salt, your blood becomes more concentrated, and your kidneys make more concentrated urine with higher salt levels to get rid of the excess sodium.

If you have normal kidneys, they can excrete up to eight hundred cubic centimeters (cc) of excess water per hour in your urine. If you drink more than a liter of water every hour, it may overwhelm your kidneys, lowering their ability to excrete water in your urine. When that happens, your kidneys dilute your urine as much as possible before reaching capacity. Any excess water begins to accumulate in your blood. When your blood contains more water than salt, it starts to get diluted. The concentration of salt in the blood slowly goes down. If you keep drinking more than a liter of water every hour for several hours, the salt concentration in your blood may get too low to sustain life, and you may die from brain swelling. Water poisoning is not very common but happens in people with psychological problems who start drinking water compulsively. Although it is not very common, water poisoning shows you how vital a good water-salt balance really is.

Similarly, if you keep eating salt without hydrating, your blood starts to get more concentrated. At first, your kidneys get rid of the excess salt by making more concentrated urine. When you eat more salt, your kidneys soon become overwhelmed, and the concentration of salt in your blood starts to go up. If you keep eating more salt, your levels can get so high that your brain ceases to function properly, and you can die. As rare as water poisoning, salt poisoning is just as deadly and shows just how important a working water-salt balance is to the body. Salt and water imbalances should be treated as soon as possible. Although food poisoning often goes away on its own, it's important to remember that it can lead to a severe water-salt imbalance.

18. Low Energy

How Hazel's Hormonal Imbalance Almost Stopped Her Heart

Learn how one important hormone regulates our body, and find out what happens when it goes up or down.

On her birthday this year, Hazel was only thirty-one years old, but she didn't feel like it. She was sleepy all the time and constantly cold. Even at home in her warm apartment, she kept several heavy sweaters on hand at all times. Everything felt like a chore, even going up and down a flight of stairs. Over the next six months, everything kept getting harder and harder for Hazel. She lost all her energy. She walked less, slept more, and only went out when it was absolutely necessary, even on warm, sunny days. Hazel was still functioning but barely.

As the weather got colder in the fall, Hazel started to feel much worse. She kept her house temperature at seventy-eight degrees, but a short trip outside could leave her shivering for hours. Even getting in and out of her car to go to work was a struggle. One afternoon after work, Hazel realized that her driveway was covered in snow. She couldn't get her car into the garage. Her husband wasn't home from work yet, and she was too tired to shovel the snow. Leaving the car parked on the side of the road, Hazel struggled slowly over the deep snowdrifts to get to her house. It was a short walk to her front door, but with each step, Hazel's boots sank deep into the snow. A full five minutes later, she reached her house.

Inside, Hazel collapsed on the couch exhausted, with her shoes and coat still on. Even inside with her winter

166

coat, she couldn't seem to get warm. She couldn't stop shivering, and each chill made her moan. She tried to get up to turn the fireplace on, but she did not have energy left to even move one leg. She lay on the couch until her husband got home from work. When he saw his wife lying on the couch, unmoving, he was worried. He touched Hazel's forehead and found it freezing. He called 911.

The paramedics arrived and started checking her vitals. Her temperature was below normal at ninety-five, as was her heart rate at forty-two. Her breathing rate was twelve per minute, and her blood pressure was 95/46. The paramedics were worried and took Hazel to the ER. On the way, they took an EKG in the ambulance and sent it to the ER doctor. The EKG showed Hazel's slow heart rate but was otherwise normal.

Something else had to be wrong. Hazel was too weak to speak, only able to answer "yes" or "no" in an inaudible whisper. Reading her lips, the paramedics managed to find out that Hazel had had no chest pain, no shortness of breath, no headaches, and no nausea or vomiting. She had been experiencing weakness and sleepiness.

At the ER, Hazel was hooked up to a heart monitor. A nurse asked Hazel's husband more questions about Hazel's condition. Hazel's husband explained that Hazel had been feeling extremely weak recently, but he'd never seen her like this. She'd been getting worse for a year, saying she didn't have the energy she used to have, but she hadn't had any health problems in the past, and she'd never been on any long-term medications.

The doctor came in and examined Hazel. He noted that her movements were slow and sluggish. He carefully listened to her heart. It was beating slowly but regularly, without skipped beats or abnormal sounds. Her lungs were clear, and her bowel sounds were slow.

Her skin was cold and dry. Her hair was thin and brittle.

"Well, I think we need to run some tests to figure out what is going on," the doctor told Hazel's husband. "The blood test results should start coming back within an hour. The rest will depend on what we find."

The nurse put a warming blanket on Hazel to warm her up since her temperature was low. She also started an IV line and drew some blood for testing.

Once the blood results started coming in, the doctor saw that Hazel's blood exhibited a lower-than-normal sodium level of 128. Hazel's kidney function was normal. Her liver and cardiac enzymes were normal as well. The doctor then ordered a TSH- (thyroid stimulating hormone) level test. As he knew, this test was an indirect measurement of thyroid-hormone activity in the body. TSH would be high when the thyroid-hormone activity was low, and TSH would be low when thyroid-hormone activity was high.

When the results of Hazel's TSH level test came back very high, the doctor noted that he had been right. Hazel's thyroid-hormone activity was very low. It was indicative, he explained to Hazel's husband, of extremely low thyroid activity.

"The thyroid," the doctor said, "is one of the very important hormones in the body that controls our metabolism. It basically controls the speed at which most of our body organs use energy. When the body releases thyroid hormones, the effect is the same as pressing down on the gas pedal in a car. Understand?"

Hazel's husband nodded.

"Energy use goes up," the doctor continued, "and output goes up. When thyroid activity is high, all the chemical activities in your organs speed up and use too much energy. Your body becomes inefficient. When thyroid activity is low, all the processes in the body slow down. I think this is what happened to Hazel. Her thyroid activity levels have probably been decreasing for a long time. Now they've reached critical levels. Her body has slowed down so much that even her heart is beating too slowly. Her body is burning so little energy that she has trouble keeping herself warm. Her brain is using so little energy that she is even having trouble thinking."

"OK, what we do now? Can we make her better? Will she be back to normal?" Hazel's husband was concerned.

"I think she will recover," the doctor said, nodding reassuringly, "with the right treatment and close monitoring. The good thing is that we have a diagnosis and know how to treat her. I am glad you brought her here before it was too late. Hazel needs to be watched very closely while we replace her thyroid hormone. We do not want to cause a rapid change in her body. We have to do it slowly and with careful heart monitoring. I think it is best if we admit Hazel to the hospital."

Hazel's husband thanked the doctor. He was so relieved that he had brought Hazel in. As he watched two nurses take his wife upstairs, he knew somehow that everything would be all right.

Upstairs, the nurses hooked Hazel up to a heart monitor and slowly started replacing her thyroid hormone. They had to watch her heart closely because there was a risk that she could develop abnormal heart rhythms during the replacement. Her body had slowly adapted to low thyroid levels, and rapid replacement could trigger problems. Watchful and meticulous, the nurses worked with Hazel's body until they had successfully increased the thyroid-hormone levels. Soon Hazel was able to go home with her husband, taking oral thyroid hormones. It got colder that winter, but Hazel felt warmer inside and out, knowing that things would be all right.

Teaching Points

Basic Approach: Slowly Developing Symptoms

As you've seen throughout *Symptoms and Diagnosis* thus far, the speed at which symptoms develop often offers clues as to what is ailing the patient. Some symptoms, like sudden blood loss, manifest instantly. Others, like rapidly progressing sepsis infections, build over a number of hours. Some are much slower, like cancerous symptoms. In this chapter, we have encountered a slowly developing hormonal imbalance that took over a year to surface.

Organ System: The Thyroid Hormone

Hormones are chemicals that regulate and fine-tune various activities inside your body. Your body has several specialized glands that make several different types of hormones. Some hormones just act on one or two organs, while others, like your thyroid, act on almost all your organs.

The thyroid hormone can be thought of as a catalyst that increases energy and activity in your body. Thyroid-hormone levels make your heart beat faster. They make you sweat more, make your muscles burn more energy, and can make you nervous, angry, or irritable. This increase in energy can eventually lead to organ damage. A heart beating too fast can develop an abnormal rhythm or simply fail. Muscles burning too much energy can cause tremors. Excessive perspiration can cause the loss of salt and water. This overall, high-energy expenditure can cause unwanted weight loss.

When your thyroid-hormone levels go down, the opposite symptoms occur. Your organs slow down, and your body slowly adapts to the low energy, which is why you may not feel too different from day to day. In today's stressful lifestyle, people attribute weakness and exhaustion to more common problems, like lack of exercise and not eating well. Sometimes these symptoms may go undetected for years before the diagnosis can be made.

What happened to Hazel is extreme, but Hazel's condition illustrates how dangerous and restrictive low thyroid levels can be. Many people go through their lives every day with low thyroid levels, blaming themselves for their exhaustion—they didn't eat enough, they ate too much, they ate the wrong food, they didn't get enough sleep, they're getting old, or they're just so stressed—never knowing that something is truly wrong. That's why it is important to get checked out if you or your loved one has been feeling like Hazel.

With a slowly developing illness like Hazel's, you need to look back and see how long you have not been feeling well. You need to compare your current state with that of last year around the same time. If you are too tired to even get out of your house this winter, and you remember going out skiing and having fun last winter, then something is really wrong. Ask your doctor about getting tested for hypothyroidism.

19. Never-Ending Complications

How Mandy Wound Up with Too Many Diagnoses

Learn to avoid falling into the trap of fictitious illness.

Mandy had been juggling a lot lately. Between a difficult divorce and a stressful, competitive, though enjoyable, job environment at an investment bank, she was under a lot of stress. On top of everything, Mandy was always worried that the anxiety she felt about her divorce would affect her performance at the bank. She'd worked hard to earn her position and the respect of everyone in her office.

Tonight when she got home, everything just felt like it was piling up. Her divorce had finally been settled, but now she was stuck with the mortgage on the house she had bought with her husband. It had depreciated in value since they had moved in, and it felt so big and empty now. Anxious, she decided to try to take her mind off of everything and do something sensible: laundry.

As she unloaded the wet clothes from the washer to the dryer, she noticed that there was a leak in the back of her washer. That was the final straw. Feeling tears coming on, she felt helpless, overwhelmed, and utterly alone. Soon she was hyperventilating. She felt as if she was choking, and her heart was pounding in her chest. As she broke out in a sweat, she called 911 and told the operator her symptoms. She described the tightness in her chest, the pounding of her heart, and the choking sensation. No, she had no chest pains, but she felt like she couldn't breathe.

The paramedics arrived at her house and found her lying on the couch with her hands on her chest. They checked her vitals, gave her baby aspirin, and took her to the ER in their ambulance.

At the ER, Mandy was triaged as a priority patient with heart-attack symptoms. A nurse hooked her up to a heart monitor, and Mandy explained what had happened.

The nurse made careful notes and then asked, "How long did the episode last?"

Mandy thought for a moment. "The worst lasted probably fifteen minutes, but I still feel like my chest is pounding."

Mandy was admitted to the hospital for observation. Throughout the night, nurses performed multiple blood tests and checked Mandy's blood pressure every four hours. She had a probe on her finger as well to monitor her blood-oxygen saturation. Lying in bed, unable to even go to the bathroom by herself because of the heart monitor, Mandy began to believe that something must seriously be wrong. She couldn't have just had a panic attack—tests would have ruled that out by now...wouldn't they? *They did so many tests*, she thought. *The chest x-ray, the EKG, all those blood tests...they'd know by now if it was nothing but a panic attack. It's so good I called 911.*

The next morning, the cardiologist came in to visit her.

"How are you feeling?" he asked.

"I am feeling much better," Mandy said, smiling. "Did I really have a heart attack?"

"Well, the admitting doctor was worried about a possible heart attack last night. That's why you were here overnight. I've just looked over all your tests, though, and I can't find any evidence of a heart attack. It could have just been a panic attack."

This should have been good news, but worry still gnawed at Mandy. She wanted to make sure she got the best treatment. Was a panic attack enough? This had felt like so much more than a panic attack.

"Well, if I didn't have a heart attack, why did I have

heart-attack symptoms?" Mandy felt the panic rising again.

"I'm not sure." The doctor shook his head. "If you want, I can order a stress test on your heart to see if you have any blocked arteries."

"Can I still have a blocked artery if I did not have a heart attack?" Mandy latched on to this.

"Well, some people do have partially blocked arteries that can cause chest pain without a heart attack," the doctor answered, cautiously. "But we don't know if that's the case here—"

"Well, don't you think we should be careful? Check every angle?" Mandy interrupted. "I think I should take the stress test."

The doctor nodded and said he'd schedule a nuclear-medicine stress test with pharmacological stress. Mandy was not to eat or drink anything until after the test was done.

"A nuclear test?" Mandy asked.

"A nuclear-medicine stress test with pharmacological—induced—stress. Basically they will inject medicine into your veins to pump your heart up, and they will take two sets of images of your heart—one at rest and one with the heart pumped. The images will show if your heart is not getting enough oxygen when it is pumped up. If your heart gets normal amounts of oxygen at rest but reduced amounts of oxygen when it is pumped up, it may suggest that you have a partial blockage. That blockage may be letting a fixed amount of blood to pass through, enough for the resting heart but not enough under stress."

Mandy nodded. This all made sense to her. Maybe her heart was not getting enough oxygen when she was stressed out. She was very glad that the doctor ordered the stress test. A few hours later, however, when the results of the stress test came back, Mandy wasn't pleased, even though the doctor had good news: The stress test had come back completely normal. There were no blockages in her arteries. Mandy could go home, the doctor said. He just wanted to see her again in one month.

"What?" Mandy asked, confused. "Are—are you sure?"

The cardiologist explained that the stress test was very sensitive to any lack of oxygen in the heart muscles. Mandy should have felt reassured, but she didn't. The doctor hadn't given her an absolute answer, yet he wanted her to go home.

"What if I have the same pain again?"

"I think it would be a good idea to come back to ER if you have chest pain again."

Two weeks later, Mandy did just that. She had the same initial symptoms, and the doctors performed more tests. When they saw she'd already had a stress test performed, however, they sent her home. All alone at home, Mandy couldn't help but feel disappointed. She needed more reassurance than this—more support and more attention. A stress test was only 85 percent accurate, the first doctor had told her—what about the other 15 percent? How could they rely on that? At least she still had her follow-up appointment to look forward to.

The day of her follow-up appointment, the cardiologist asked about Mandy's second ER visit.

"Well, it was almost like the first time," Mandy said. She felt a release as she described her episode. It felt good to talk to someone about what bothered her. Since her divorce, she'd tried to put on a brave face at work. Not sharing anything with her coworkers was isolating. "I had that pressure-like pain, and I felt like I could not breathe. I have been so worried because I know you mentioned a fifteen percent chance of blockage. The ER doctor was so dismissive, though, Doctor. I'm glad for this follow-up."

The doctor studied Mandy.

"Mandy, I don't think you have a blockage either. The EKG and blood tests done in the ER look normal—"

"So you're saying you're absolutely sure I don't have a blockage?" Mandy broke in, fixing the doctor with an anxious stare.

"I can't say anything absolutely, Mandy," the doctor said slowly, "but I think a blockage is unlikely—"

Mandy interrupted again.

"Of course you can be one hundred percent sure— there must be a way. I've had a terrible year, and I can't afford to suffer like this. Surely there must be a test you can do." Mandy finished and waited anxiously.

The doctor sighed.

"There's a procedure we can do, but it's very invasive and unnecessary. It's called a cardiac cath. We would insert a catheter through your groin and push it all the way to your heart while looking at it under the x-ray screen. We would inject a dye into your heart arteries and look directly for any blockages. It's the most accurate test we have, but I wouldn't recommend it. It has risks."

"I am willing to take those risks, Doctor. You can't know what I've been through this year. I can't stand not knowing, wondering, and worrying."

The doctor was reluctant, but he also didn't want Mandy to feel as if she wasn't being heard. He advised her to go home but to come back to the ER if the chest pain came back. He would do the cardiac catheterization himself at that time if Mandy really needed it.

One week later, Mandy felt the chest pain again. She went to ER. As promised, an ER doctor called the cardiologist and took her to the cath lab. Mandy was relieved. She was finally feeling taken care of. The nurse in the cath lab was very kind. She gently prepared Mandy for the procedure, cleaning and shaving her skin at her groin near the catheter entry point. She changed Mandy into a clean patient gown and showed her a video of how the procedure was done. Mandy was very impressed with the way the lab was set up. Everyone seemed so organized and attentive. She definitely felt like she was in good hands.

On the cath table, after an injection to help her relax, Mandy was happy for the first time in months. She was finally getting the attention and care that she needed. Later, in the recovery room, the doctor assured her that she had no blockages. Mandy was finally relieved. She'd gotten the reassurance she needed. She went home feeling relaxed and a little less lonely.

A few weeks passed. The stress at Mandy's job increased again, and at the end of the day, her house seemed bigger and emptier than ever. Her mortgage felt heavier. She started having pain again. At first, it almost cheered her up—perhaps it was time to go back to the ER and to the cath lab. She hadn't felt alone there. But the pain was mild, she realized, and only located in her stomach. If only she had a reason to go back to the ER. If only she could feel cared for again. Slowly, Mandy began to worry that the pain in her stomach might be something serious. She did some research on stomach pain—she couldn't go to the ER uninformed. What if she needed surgery? She thought of the peace she had felt in the cath lab again. She probably did need surgery—her Internet research had raised the possibility of gallbladder problems. What if she needed it removed? Mandy was disappointed when she read that gallbladder issues manifest in the upper right side of the stomach. She didn't have pain there. Or did she? Over the next few days, the pain seemed to migrate to the right side of her abdomen. At least when she thought about it, it did.

177

Mandy knew just what to do. She went back to the ER and recited all the symptoms of gallbladder pain and infection she had absorbed in her research. Based on her textbook description of gallbladder problems, the ER doctor ordered an ultrasound of Mandy's gallbladder.

Once again, Mandy's results came back normal. Once again, Mandy felt empty and disappointed. She went home and began researching gallbladder pain again. She read that in a small number of cases, people could have gallbladder pain despite having a normal-looking gall bladder. She just needed to have persistent and convincing symptoms. After several ER visits over the next few weeks with more and more refined symptoms, she was finally able to convince a surgeon that she had a-calculus cholecystitis, a rare inflammation of the gallbladder without gallstones. Normally gallstones cause the inflammation in the gallbladder, but in some cases, the pain and inflammation could manifest without visible stones. She went back to the surgeon with her theory and finally had her gallbladder removed. What a relief it was to be so taken care of, to know that she wasn't alone. What a relief to know that surgery could solve emotional as well as physical problems.

Over the next several years, whenever Mandy was struggling emotionally, medical illnesses seemed to manifest as well. After thorough Internet research, she was always able to find her symptoms, even if they didn't always match up initially. At the ER, she would exaggerate or manipulate her symptoms to match the condition with which she had diagnosed herself. She knew now from past experience that doctors didn't always know what she needed. Sometimes they needed that extra push.

Again and again, Mandy convinced her doctors that she needed surgery. Soon she had multiple scars in her abdomen from surgeries for phantom illnesses. She developed a legitimate bowel obstruction secondary to adhesion related to her many unnecessary surgeries. This required necessary medical treatment. Despite the fact that she was hurting herself by trying to heal herself, she always managed to have surgery every few months.

Years passed this way until the day a new doctor reviewed her chart for a new symptom and became suspicious of Mandy's medical history. It was peppered with ER visits and multiple surgeries. As he looked at the paper trail of Mandy's medical records, he noticed a pattern. Except for the bowel obstruction that resulted from postsurgery adhesion, there was no evidence for Mandy's other ailments and no test results that suggested Mandy would have needed all the surgeries she had undergone. That very first procedure, the cardiac catheterization, had been completely normal. The testing of Mandy's gallbladder after removal revealed no actual inflammation, just as her appendix showed no inflammation after the appendectomy. Something was wrong with Mandy, the doctor realized, but the symptoms led to a diagnosis that Mandy would never come up with on her own.

The doctor asked Mandy how she ended up having so many surgeries. She recoiled instantly, suspicious. Did this doctor doubt how difficult all this was for her? She became uncommunicative, but the doctor had all the information he needed. He realized that Mandy's surgeries followed the pattern consistent with factitious disorder or Munchausen syndrome. Unfortunately, before he could establish the diagnosis, Mandy left the hospital and never returned. The next time she began to feel the need for surgery again, she went to another hospital on the other side of town that was operated by a separate health-care system.

Teaching Points

Basic Approach: When to Let Go

Throughout *Symptoms and Diagnosis* you have learned about the importance of communicating with your doctor and of working together to find a diagnosis. Sometimes you have to be insistent. Sometimes you have to trust your instincts, even when they differ from your doctor's. It's important to do your own research and to raise questions about diagnoses. This is what I have told my patients throughout my medical career, and it's one of the most important messages I hope you take away from reading this book.

That being said, you must be aware of the limitations of current medical diagnostic technologies. Not every symptom has a physical diagnosis. So how do you know when you need to pursue a diagnosis and when you need to let it go? Listen to your body, not your mind.

Organ System: The Psychology of Illness

As in Mandy's case, sometimes the mind lies to the body. When you're dealing with a lot of emotional stress, it can manifest physically. It's always important to get physical symptoms checked out, but it's also important to understand when unexplained symptoms are emotional. Unexplained symptoms can be frustrating. Unfortunately modern medical practice can't always explain every symptom. It is designed to do everything in its power, however, to make sure that something important is not overlooked. While your doctor may consider many diagnoses during the examination process, most diagnoses are eliminated one by one. This process of ruling out illnesses is necessary, but it can have a significant impact on the patient, who may have difficulty accepting the fact that after all the testing and observation, the diagnosis is "none of the above." Ruling out a disease may be reassuring to a doctor, but it can be stressful for a patient. It can even lead the patient to distrust the doctor.

It is unclear how most patients develop Munchausen syndrome, but our medical system is certainly not designed to detect such patients. It is, in fact, very easy for a patient suffering from Munchausen syndrome to game the system and seek unnecessary treatment and procedures. When a patient reports symptoms manufactured to mislead a doctor, he or she tampers with the most important diagnostic tool a doctor has: communication.

When patients fall into this vicious cycle of Munchausen syndrome, they forget why, when, and how it was triggered. They fake their symptoms to no material benefit. Their only motive is to get the unnecessary treatment or procedure because it gives them satisfaction in doing so and to receive attention and care. It is very difficult to treat those patients once they are on this path. That's why it's so important to seek mental-health counseling if you suspect that you or a loved one are going down this path. If a loved one is under a lot of stress, you need to watch him or her very carefully when he or she goes through the medical system. In today's society, it is easier and more acceptable to seek medical attention for physical symptoms than for mental symptoms, but it is best to seek and address any mental-health issues before the mind starts blaming the body.

20. Open Your Eyes

How Howard's Doctors Thought He Would Never Wake Up from a Coma

Learn how doctors investigate a coma and test human brain function.

The ER doctor walked slowly around Howard's hospital bed, mentally scratching his head. Howard's case was very unusual. A thirty-year-old unconscious male brought to the ER by police, Howard was breathing normally and his heart rate was fine, but he was completely unresponsive. He appeared to be in a coma.

The doctor asked the police what had happened and how they had found him. He hoped their description of the events leading up to Howard's admittance to the ER would reveal some key to Howard's condition.

It had started with a hit-and-run call. Someone had seen Howard rear-end someone on the highway ramp and then back up and speed off. Once the police spotted Howard's car based on the caller's description of said car and license plate, they attempted to pull Howard over, but he sped up, leading the police on a car chase for a good fifteen minutes. Turning onto a rural road, Howard headed toward an open barn. When the police closed in on him, Howard got out of his car and took off on foot. The police followed but couldn't find Howard initially. It took them twenty minutes to discover his body on the ground around the side of the barn. He was lying on his back, completely unresponsive. They were able to secure Howard and have him checked out by medics, who recommended they bring their runaway patient to the ER.

"Did you find any drugs or alcohol in his car or on his person?" the doctor asked.

"Nope," one policeman answered, shaking his head. "The car was clean—no drugs, alcohol, or prescription pills. He only had his wallet on him."

The doctor thanked the police officer and turned back to examining Howard. He looked at Howard's eyes and called his name several times. He shook him by the shoulder, but even then, Howard did not move or respond.

"I am sorry," the doctor said loudly to Howard, "but I need to examine your eyes." He forced Howard's eyes open. The pupils were of a normal size. They responded normally to light. He could not find anything abnormal.

The doctor listened to Howard's heart. It was beating regularly without a single skipped beat. Howard's lungs sounded normal as well, and he was breathing without any problems. The doctor detected no bruises or signs of injury anywhere on Howard's body.

"Howard, will you lift up your left leg please?" the doctor asked loudly.

No response.

"Howard, can you wiggle your toes please?"

Again no response.

"Howard, can you squeeze my fingers please?"

Still there was no response. The doctor proceeded with his exam.

"Howard, I will now pinch your legs a little bit to see if they will move. I am not trying to hurt you."

The nurse came into the room, frowning. "So what do you think?" she asked.

"Well, I don't really know. His vitals are normal, but he is not responding at all as you can see. I see no evidence of trauma. I'd like some routine blood tests, a CT scan of his head, and…a drug test."

The nurse alerted the blood lab and the radiology department. The lab drew blood and started an IV line for Howard. He didn't respond to the needles or to the

Foley catheter inserted to drain his urine for the test. There was no movement or indication of registered pain. The doctor moved Howard's arms and legs and met no resistance. It seemed as though Howard did not have any control over his limbs.

Nurses slowly wheeled Howard to the CT scan room. It took four of them to lay his limp body in the machine. The scan was quick, as Howard lay completely motionless. The technician did not have to say his usual phrase, "Hold still for just a minute please."

While the doctor was waiting for the blood tests to come back, he couldn't resist pulling up the CT scan on his computer. Examining the images several times, frame by frame, he was still unable to spot any abnormality. The patient had a normal brain, and there was no bleeding, no swelling, and no sign of a stroke. Howard seemed absolutely fine. So what was wrong?

The urine test result was the first to come back, showing small traces of marijuana and cocaine. The nurse handed over the piece of paper with the drug-screen result to the doctor.

"Do you think this is what caused all this?" she asked.

"Well, it looks like he did use some marijuana and cocaine recently, but that's not why he's in a coma. This doesn't look like a cocaine overdose—his heart rate is normal and his blood pressure has been very good. You cannot have a cocaine overdose with a normal heart rate and normal blood pressure like Howard's. My guess is he used it sometime in the last few days. It's not really affecting him at this point."

"Then what do you think it is?"

"I am still baffled myself," the doctor said, shaking his head.

The rest of the blood work came back normal. Howard had normal levels of blood glucose, thyroid hormone, sodium, and potassium in his blood. His liver and kidney functions were all normal too.

"Well, I don't have any diagnosis of his coma. Can you get the admitting doctor on the phone? Howard needs to be admitted to the hospital for observation. Maybe they can figure something out upstairs."

"Sounds like a good idea to me," the nurse said, agreeing.

Once admitted, a neurologist thoroughly examined Howard. He started his evaluation the same way the ER doctor did, but he went through several more steps. After Howard did not respond to arm and leg pinches, the neurologist gently opened both his eyelids and asked him to look up, look down, and look to the sides. Howard's eyeballs did not move at all. It was as if they were looking at a fixed target in the distance. The doctor then closed his patient's eyelids and pushed firmly above the top of the eyes, looking closely to see if any of the muscles in Howard's face moved, but they did not. Howard did not even show the slightest sign of a grimace under such firm pressure.

For the next part of his evaluation, the neurologist brought in a medical student. He would need extra help to perform this test.

"Joan, thank you for agreeing to assist me in conducting a caloric testing and doll's-eye testing on Howard today. Can you tell me what you know about caloric testing in this type of situation?"

"Yes, Doctor. In this type of situation, caloric testing is used to test brain-stem function. If reflexes register, then the brain stem is functioning. If they are absent, it is not."

"Very good. Let's get started with the doll's-eye reflex first. Can you keep his eyelids open while I move his head from side to side? Look carefully and note what his eyeballs do when I move his head."

The neurologist moved Howard's head to the right. Howard's eyeballs initially moved with his head but then wandered a little bit and moved slightly to the left. The neurologist moved Howard's head to the left. The eyes moved with the head and stayed there for a little while and slowly moved back and forth and finally moved to the right.

"OK, Joan, what do you think?"

"I think this is inconclusive. I think we did see some reflex movement, but it was not as clear-cut as we expected. Let's proceed to the caloric testing and see what happens."

"Good thinking. Let's do that. Please inject the water. I will watch his eye movement."

Joan fitted the syringe with a short flexible tube and filled it with cold water. She pushed the tube all the way inside Howard's right ear until it reached the eardrum. The neurologist opened both the eyelids and looked carefully at the eyeballs. Joan then slowly injected the cold water into Howard's right ear. His eyeballs moved to the left.

Joan took the syringe out, waited for five minutes, and repeated the same procedure in the left ear. This time, Howard's eyes moved to the right.

"So what do you think now?"

"I think we just saw some definitive evidence that the brain-stem reflex is still intact, but I am not sure why the doll's test was not that definitive."

"That's correct, Joan. I'm not sure either what the doll's-eye test results mean. We still need to complete a thorough workup. I will start with an electroencephalogram first."

They took him to the EEG room and placed several electrodes on his head. Those electrodes were connected to a monitor that would record the electrical activity in Howard's brain. The electrodes measured different wave patterns at different frequencies. When the neurologist looked at those waves, he could not identify any abnormal patterns. It was no different from a random EEG taken of a normal, conscious person's brain. He had the usual mixture of different frequencies, and there was nothing in the brain waves that suggested a seizure or an abnormal finding.

After the EEG failed to provide any answers, the neurologist decided to order an MRI of Howard's brain. The MRI would give him a much better picture of the brain than the CT scan alone could provide. A nurse prepared Howard for the MRI, making sure he had no metal on him and that his IV lines were set. Afterward, the neurologist looked at the MRI images carefully and analyzed them frame by frame. Everything appeared perfectly normal. After reviewing all the tests that had been done in the hospital, the neurologist could not point to any nonfocal symptoms, which is to say that he could not pinpoint any particular portion of the brain responsible for Howard's state. He determined that Howard's symptoms were not caused by any neurological problems. Some other organ system must have been affecting Howard's brain.

Once the neurologist had ruled out neurological issues, the medical doctors at the hospital were left with no choice but to provide Howard with supportive care and watch him closely. He was still breathing normally, and his heart was still beating regularly. However, he was not waking up to eat, drink, or relieve himself. They started some basic supportive treatment to take care of his nutrition and his excretion, including an IV nutrition regimen that included sugars, protein, fats, vitamins, and minerals in soluble form. The vitamin drip was designed to take care of Howard's immediate nutritional needs.

They also placed a Foley catheter in his bladder so that they could continuously drain his urine. He would not suffer from bladder dissension and leakage from not being awake or being aware of needing to urinate.

Three days passed. The doctors still could not determine the cause of Howard's coma. With the nutritional and other supportive care in place, his body was still not functioning normally, but his brain reflexes remained active. He still did not respond at all. They tested several new theories each day. They sent his blood to specialized labs to test for all types of uncommon and highly specialized chemicals and drugs that could potentially cause Howard's coma.

On the fourth day, the neurologist got a call from a very excited nurse. It was the nurse taking care of Howard. She told the doctor that the patient had suddenly woken up and asked for food. The doctor ran to Howard's room and started asking him questions, but Howard was in no mood to talk to the doctor. He wanted something to eat. The doctor had the nurse quickly check Howard's vital signs. Everything was within normal limits, and Howard could safely eat something. He asked the nurse to order a meal right away.

When the food arrived, Howard started eating very quickly. After eating steadily for some time, Howard finally began to talk. He revealed that he had actually been awake the entire time. He just hadn't wanted to talk to the police.

"Let me get this straight. You were faking a coma?" The doctor was shocked. He thought of all the tests Howard had gone through.

"Yeah," Howard said between bites of mashed potato. "I was. Like I told you, I was trying to get away from the police."

"Howard, the tests we gave you were very painful. We flushed cold and hot water in your ears and pried your eyes open. How could you go through all that and not even blink?"

"I guess I have a very high tolerance for torture, Doc." Howard took a gulp of water and started back in on the potatoes. "My dad was an addict. He beat me all the time when I was young. He overdosed when I was twelve, though. I've also been in and out of psych hospitals since I was a kid. I'm bipolar, and I used to be on a bunch of drugs. I stopped taking them, though, five years ago. They made my head all cloudy. A little cocaine plus a little weed balances me out now more than any pharmaceuticals ever did."

"Howard," the doctor began, "would you characterize your behavior as balanced? You caused a car accident and fled the scene. How much cocaine do you use?"

"Oh, that." Howard shrugged. "Not much. I just use a little bit on the weekends. Normally I just stick to weed during the week."

"If you could tolerate the pain from all those tests, Howard, what made you decide to break your coma and come out?"

"I was starving, Doc."

The neurologist was surprised. Of course Howard hadn't been eating. His IV drip had been enough to sustain him but not enough to curb his appetite. After this realization, the medical mystery of this case was solved. Howard had been in a psychogenic coma, a rare dissociative state triggered by upsetting events, mostly seen in patients suffering from depression, bipolar disorder, or schizophrenia.

Teaching Points

Basic Approach: Wakefulness and Consciousness

Your brain is a very complicated organ. It not only controls your thoughts and emotions but also your movement, your balance, and your senses. It even controls wakefulness and consciousness. In effect, your brain directs your body. It can even shut your body down when you have problems with awareness or with wakefulness and arousal.

When you have problems with awareness, you are unable to hear or feel anything around you. Your brain cannot process any external signals and you are not aware of your surroundings. In the most intense unaware state, you are designated as vegetative. In a vegetative state, you may lose awareness while maintaining normal levels of arousal or wakefulness because awareness and arousal are processed in two different areas of the brain. Awareness or consciousness are processed in the higher brain center, where thoughts and memories are processed. Wakefulness or arousal are processed in the lower brain center near the brain stem, where signals from the higher brain pass through the neck and down to the spine. Wakefulness can vary from fully awake to complete coma. Someone with damage in the higher brain center but with a normal lower brain center may appear fully awake but may not have awareness of anything in his or her environment.

Technically a patient in a coma has a disorder that affects wakefulness, not consciousness. You can think of a coma as a deep, deep sleep. A very heavy sleeper takes a lot of stimuli to wake up—shouting, alarms, or shaking. A coma is a much deeper sleep, one that can be caused by two different problems: issues with the lower brain center (the brain stem) or widespread issues affecting the whole brain. Since the brain stem controls wakefulness, brain-stem dysfunction causes a deep coma with other subtle signs of brain-stem dysfunction. A coma caused by dysfunction throughout the brain is different and is usually caused by widespread problems affecting the whole body.

Organ System: The Brain and the Mind

Although the brain is immensely complex, there are some simple nerve pathways in the brain that can be tested. These tests essentially act as simple circuit tests like those one might run on electrical wiring. When you flip a switch on a lamp and the bulb lights up, it means that the path of electricity from the power source to the light bulb is still intact. A brain function test works in a similar way, with testing cranial nerves coming out of the brain and supplying innervation to the organs in your head. These cranial nerves act as circuit testers for different regions of the brain, creating different muscle reactions when we test them.

Pupil reactions to light, eyeball movement, facial muscular movement, and tongue movement are a few reactions governed by these cranial nerves that we can test. Each is linked to a different part of the brain. Failure of one of these areas to react to testing points to dysfunction in a particular part of the brain.

When testing a patient in coma, it is important to find out if the coma is caused by a problem in the brain stem. Brain-stem function is tested in two ways: the doll's-eye test and caloric testing. In a doll's-eye test, the doctor moves the patient's head from side to side while keeping the patient's eyes open. If the pathways of nerves passing through the brain stem are intact, the eyes will move in the opposite direction of the head movement. The doll's-eye test only works on a comatose patient, since a conscious patient can fix his or her eyes and look anywhere he or she wishes to. In caloric testing, doctors inject cold and warm water into the patient's eardrums. If the patient's brain stem is intact, it produces a certain type of eye movement. In hindsight, the doll's-eye test produced inconclusive results in Howard's case because Howard was not truly comatose. He was suppressing his eye movements voluntarily to simulate a coma.

Howard's story demonstrates quite keenly that the

patient's role in reaching a diagnosis is just as important as the doctor's. By helping (or not helping) his or her doctor, the patient provides key information that all the modern technology and detailed scientific knowledge in the world cannot provide. The most advanced equipment and medical tests couldn't show the neurologist that Howard was faking his symptoms. Tests can only help confirm or invalidate background information and hypotheses. Technology used in imaging and testing can only be used in the context of the patient's symptoms. If a patient appears comatose and the MRI comes back normal, the doctor cannot determine the cause of the coma. He or she can only determine that the coma is not caused by structural brain damage.

As you've learned throughout *Symptoms and Diagnosis*, getting the right diagnosis requires equal cooperation from the doctor and patient. While there are thousands of books that teach doctors to become better diagnosticians, there are very few books like this one, which help patients communicate better with doctors to nail down an accurate diagnosis. I hope this book has helped you better understand how medical diagnoses are reached and how important your role is in achieving them.

Made in the USA
Columbia, SC
23 December 2017